Mona Jawad
Michael Pfaffenberger
811 New York Ave
Brooklyn, New York

The ER Intern Pocket Survival Guide

Todd C. Rothenhaus, M.D.
Thomas M. Masterson, M.D.

Former Interns
The George Washington University Medical Center
Washington, D.C.

Other titles from International Medical Publishing

The Intern Pocket Survival Guide
The CCU Intern Pocket Survival Guide
The Surgical Intern Pocket Survival Guide
The ICU Intern Pocket Survival Guide
The Oncology Intern Pocket Survival Guide

The EKG Pocket Survival Guide
The ACLS Pocket Survival Guide
The PALS Pocket Survival Guide

The Pocket Guide to Eponyms and Subtle Signs of Disease
How to be a Truly Excellent Junior Medical Student

Clinician's Handbook of Preventive Services
Guide to Clinical Preventive Services, 2nd edition
First Aid

Sixth Printing.

The ER Intern Pocket Survival Guide.

This title is available from your Bayer pharmaceutical representative
Other titles are available mail order from:
International Medical Publishing, Inc.
13017 Wisteria Drive, #313
Germantown, MD 20874

Published by International Medical Publishing, Inc.
101 Pommander Walk
Alexandria, Virginia 22314
703-519-0807

ISBN 0-9634063-2-9.

Printed in U.S.A.

Preface

"Honesty of purpose and determination to succeed stand out in a physician's attitude and create confidence and hope. Obviously, half-hearted vacillation creates doubt and anxiety." Austen Fox Riggs, MD 1929.

Even to the most seasoned physician, managing multiple patients, many of whom are quite sick, is challenging. Without experience, doing it well is nearly impossible.

This book is aimed at interns beginning their rotation in the emergency department. It is a guide to the workup of the most common complaints. While most books are written to be used after getting the H&P, this book is meant to be read before seeing the patient. Examine the contents and read the introductory pages before your first shift.

Problems in this book are presented alphabetically. A few common pediatric problems are discussed. An antibiotic book as well as a drug reference will complement this guide. More elaborate references and senior help should always be close at hand.

In an ED with good nurses, therapy is often initiated before you see the patient. While this is good for patient care, it isn't good for your training. To this end, much of this book concerns what to do before saying hello.

Therapeutics suggested are just that-suggestions. Please consult an attending or resident when you find yourself seeing, doing, or ordering something for the first time.

Physicians who have particularly influenced us are Drs. Hunt, Scott, Smith, and Edlich. We thank them for their tutelage. We are especially grateful to Dr. Yolanda Haywood for her editorial assistance. The opinions expressed are solely ours.

This book is dedicated to Clinton Shipp.

THE AUTHORS

Hospitals

"All parts of the metropolis discover, at every turn, large buildings of splendid elevation fitted up in a style of grandeur, not to say elegance, quite unsuited to the rational demands of the humbler classes that throng them daily."
Building News, May 15, 1857.

"A hospital may be likened to a hive. What gives it character is not its queen, but its workers."
Harvey Cushing, MD 1928.

"If poverty is an evil, or disease a misfortune, then certainly, where they coexist, the miseries of each are intensified by the presence of the other, and the sum total is multiplied an hundred fold. And as the political economists have not yet succeeded in finding any means for preventing pauperism,— nor the physicians, in discovering any method of wholly annihilating disease,— it follows that society must still continue to provide for those of its members who are, by either or both of these calamities, incapacitated from taking care of themselves."
Henry G. Clark, "Outlines of a Plan for a Free City Hospital." 1860.

Contents

The Laws of Internship

1. Listen when nature calls.

2. Make time for meals.

3. Sleep whenever possible.

4. Call spouse or significant other when on call.

Approach to the Patient in the Emergency Department

Attending: *"What have you been doing in there?"*
Student: *"Getting the history."*
Attending: *"But he can't talk."*
Student: *"That's why it took so long."*

The traditional approach to medical problem solving is history, physical, labs, studies, assessment, plan, therapy. The hallmark of emergency medicine, and what makes it difficult for novices, is rapid assessment and initiation of therapy frequently before any history is obtained.

The approach to all patients in the ED should be an quick initial survey of ABCs and vital signs, followed by a brief assessment and institution of initial measures. This approach (1) makes it less likely that a patient will crash without warning, (2) allows you to leave that patient unattended if your attention becomes needed elsewhere, and (3) speeds things up.

Obviously, if a patient can say "Hi Doc, I feel terrible," he has probably passed the ABCs (although he may not be able to in ten minutes). Remember, if you get stuck anywhere in the ABCs you can't go on—an IV does little good in a patient who is not breathing.

What follows is a brief discussion on how its done. Get senior residents and attendings on board when things get sticky.

For your own safety:

1. Hepatitis series.
2. Seasonal flu-shot.
3. Rubella titer.
4. PPD per annum.
5. Universal precautions.

Airway

"Our main business is not to see what lies dimly at a distance, but to do what lies clearly at hand." Thomas Carlyle.

The most common cause of airway obstruction is the tongue falling back into the posterior pharynx from poor airway reflexes. Other causes of airway compromise include vomit, blood, laryngeal edema, foreign body, trauma and tumors.

When airway problems strike:

1. Verify obstruction: look, listen, and feel for breaths. Sitting upright (tripod), drooling and stridor are bad -- get help!
2. Establish an adequate airway with the triple airway maneuver:
   Tilt head backward, except in cases of suspected C-spine injury.
   Thrust jaw forward with fingers behind both rami of the mandible.
   Open mouth using thumbs to retract the lower lips.
3. Summon assistance.
4. Suction secretions and perform finger sweep if necessary.
5. Insert the proper adjunctive airway:

Nasal Airway: used in obtunded or semi-comatose patients who still have a partial gag reflex. It keeps the tongue from falling back onto the base of the posterior pharynx. The flange on the end prevents it from sliding all the way into the nose. Insert it into the larger nostril, parallel to the floor of the nasal cavity, with the tapered end upward. After it makes the turn and passes downward, gently rotate it to assume its natural curvature.

Oral Airway: causes gagging in patients with even minimal airway reflexes. Do not allow it to be used as a bite block for awake patients who have been intubated. Insert it using a tongue blade, upside down initially, then rotate it to depress the tongue downward.

6. Provide O_2.
7. An Endotracheal Tube is the definitive airway. Once a patient is intubated:
   Listen over the epigastrium for gastric insufflation.
   Listen over both lung fields for equal breath sounds.
   Check end-tidal CO_2 with detector.
   Insert NGT.
   Call for stat PCXR and ventilator.

Breathing

Once an adequate airway is established, breathing must be reassessed. Patients with depressed mental status may not ventilate sufficiently.

1. Reassess adequacy of respiration: *look, listen* and *feel.*

2. Provide ventilatory assistance as needed using the bag-valve-mask: to obtain the best seal, keep the middle, ring, and little fingers of both hands around both angles of the mandible and pull the mandible upward. Hold the mask on the face with both thumbs and index fingers around the mask in a "C" fashion and let an assistant squeeze the bag. Alternatively, keep the dominant hand on the patient and squeeze the bag with the non-dominant hand.

3. If the patient is intubated, pull off the mask and attach the bag to the ET tube directly. Bag about 15 times a minute.

Circulation

Circulation is assessed with pulses and blood pressure. A good rule of thumb is as follows:

Radial pulse palpable	SBP > 80
Femoral pulse palpable	SBP > 70
Carotid pulse palpable	SBP > 60

Remember that BP can be normal in the face of exsanguinating hemorrhage. Orthostatics need to be performed if hypovolemia is suspected. The Doppler is often necessary to auscultate a faint BP and is reported as the pressure at which sounds are first heard (systolic). Be a bit cautious about treating aberrations that arise with automated cuffs.

Capillary refill and coolness or clamminess are important, subtle, clues of inadequate tissue perfusion. See shock/hypotension page 59.

If no pulse is obtainable, initiate cardiac compressions:

1. Move to the patients side and place the heel of one hand over the lower half of the sternum, two finger-widths above the xiphoid. Place the opposite hand above the first.

2. Compress downward (1.5-2cm in adults) holding downward for 50% of the cycle and releasing for 50%. Don't lift your hands off the patient.

3. Compress 80-100 times per minute. Coordinate respirations as follows:
   - 15 compressions for every 2 manual breaths if working alone.
   - 5 compressions per single inflation if someone else is bagging.
   - 80-100 uncoordinated compressions per minute if intubated.

Vital Signs

"1. Get the facts. 2. Analyze the facts. 3. Arrive at a decision-and then act on that decision."
Dale Carnegie.

Vital signs are frequently the only objective "numbers" you will obtain on a patient. Check the vitals before sitting down to talk to a patient and comment on (or copy) them to make sure you have noted them. Revitalize any patient who's vitals are abnormal, and avoid discharging patients with abnormal vital signs without commenting on them on the chart or addressing them in follow up-i.e. primary care follow up for mild HTN.

Weight and Vital Signs by Age:

Age	Wt(kg)	HR	Resp	SBP	DBP
Newborn	1	145	<40	40-60	20-36
Newborn	2-3	125	<40	50-70	30-45
1 month	4	120	24-35	64-96	30-62
6 months	7	130	24-35	60-118	50-70
1 year	10	130	20-30	66-126	41-91
2-3 years	12-14	120	20-30	74-124	39-89
4-5 years	16-18	100	20-30	79-119	45-85
6-8 yrs	20-26	100	12-25	80-124	45-85
10-12 yrs	32-42	75	12-25	85-135	55-88
>14	>50	70	12-18	90-140	60-90
Adult	70	70	12-16	90-140	60-90

Initial Measures

Once the ABCs are tackled, consider initial therapy and monitoring techniques.

- Oxygen
- IV access & labs
- Fluids
- Finger stick
- Medications
    - Nebs
    - Furosemide
    - Naloxone
    - Nitrates
    - Glucose
    - Morphine

- Type and Cross
- Cardiac Monitor
- Pulse-oximeter
- External pacer paddles
- EKG
- Stat X-rays

History

"I keep six honest-serving men (they taught me all I know); their names are what and why and when and how and where and who."
Rudyard Kipling.

Target your H&P towards what brought the patient in.
If a patient says "I feel like I'm going to die," take him or her very seriously.

Patients with multiple diseases and medications always seem to arrive without family or documentation, and much of the ED history needs to be obtained from people other than the patient. For accidents, find out from rescue personnel the condition at the scene. For medical patients brought in by ambulance, paramedics often have a tremendous amount of information to relay; talk to them directly if you can. Family and friends usually know something about chronic conditions and medications, and phone calls are often helpful. Give medical records a try, your patient may have been through the hospital before.

For simple problems like lacerations and fractures, use the pneumonic AMPLE: Allergies, Medications, PMH, Last meal, Event.

Direct the ROS toward the differential diagnosis-e.g. for the patient with CP inquire about cardiac, pulmonary, or GI symptoms. Ask specifically about CAD, PUD, HTN, and DM in every patient. Inquire about immunizations in children.

Be sure to document repeat visits for the same complaint, and treat repeat visitors with a high degree of scrutiny.

Document your history as soon as you are through with it.

Physical

Inexperienced physicians focus on the obvious injury or complaint, and often miss the big picture. Make sure to cover the ABCs first, then look specifically for associated injuries or conditions e.g. if the foot is injured in a fall, check the spine; if a patient has cardiac ischemia, consider GI bleed.

Some general rules apply:

1. Vitals, mental status, and general appearance are part of every physical. Physical exams are hard to do unless the patient is *undressed.*

2. All trauma patients deserve a complete head to toe examination after ABCs have been addressed.

3. All medical patients deserve a heart, lung, abdomen and back exam in addition to any organ systems involved.

4. A good neurologic exam consists of (i) cranial nerves (ii) cerebellar exam (iii) motor (iv) sensory (v) reflexes and (vi) mental status.

5. Document your physical as soon as you are finished with it.

6. Avoid the description "drunk" in favor of the observation "odor of alcohol on breath."

ED Diagnostics

"Charges are not costs." Phillip Birnbaum, Ph.D.

1. Justify each test by asking how it will change your management.
2. Tests to rule out serious disease are valuable even if negative.
3. The radiology resident has difficulty with #2.
4. Order only what will help you at the moment.
5. Don't order tests that no one will follow up on.
6. If a test is necessary, order it regardless of cost.
7. Get a consult or attending input before ordering big ticket items.
8. Non-determinate is not negative.

ED Therapeutics

"The ultimate aim of quality control is to build popularity, for without it, sales and profits lag." Tom Miner.

1. Does the patient really need an IV?
2. Does the patient require fluids?
3. Could that IV medication be PO?
4. Any chance the patient is pregnant?
5. Is my therapy working, or is the patient getting worse?
6. Is my patient in pain?
7. Did I pull up the side rails after the physical?
8. When did I last see my patient, i.e. don't leave patients for hours without checking on them?
9. Did I tell the patient about the test I ordered?

Disposition

"Can I get a cab pass?"

1. Have you excluded the worst?
2. Have you talked to the patient's private physician?
3. Can the patient walk?
4. Does the patient understand the discharge instructions?
5. Can the patient read?
6. Can she afford to fill the prescription?
7. Can the patient take care of herself?
8. Will the patient follow up?
9. Would it be better to admit the patient?
10. Does the admitting team understand the problem?
11. Why hasn't that patient been taken upstairs yet?

Shifts

"I said in my heart, I am sick of four walls and a ceiling. I have need of the sky. I have business with the grass." Richard Hovey, 1896.

Sign in:

1. Jot down a "scut" list.

2. Make "walk-rounds."

3. If your ED has a board that indicates who is seeing a particular patient, write in your name.

4. Make sure the person going off has filled out all the appropriate parts of the chart.

5. If any patients are ready to be admitted and phone calls need to be made, make sure they get done before the person going off leaves.

6. You should know and agree with the diagnoses of the patients you will send home no matter who worked them up.

Sign out:

1. Go over each patient with the oncoming intern or resident. Be sure to give the name, chief complaint, brief history, physical and probable diagnoses. List outstanding tests and whatever else might be keeping the patient in the ED.

2. Phone in any admissions you have.

3. Give yourself ten minutes to finish charts and procedures.

4. If you have particular ideas about discharge instructions, fill them in.

5. Leave. You'll be back again all to soon.

Charts

The now old medicolegal aphorism states: "if you didn't chart it, it didn't happen." While this presents a hassle, consider who else reads the chart:

1. The attending, who is ultimately responsible for the patient.
2. Consultants, who often read the chart rather than bothering you.
3. The next ED physician who takes care of the patient (when he returns for the same problem).
4. Billing, who use the chart to help your hospital get paid.
5. Lawyers, whose existence is barely justified.

Difficult Patients

Quite often patients come to the emergency room in the middle of the night with complaints that seem trivial. Many have seen another physician for the same condition, and come to the ED for a fresh opinion or because they were dissatisfied with their treatment. Still others arrive and get triaged for one complaint but go on to report a lengthy string of positives on their review of systems.

There is little use asking a patient who comes in with a trivial complaint why he or she decided to come in to the emergency room in the middle of the night, but be aware of hidden agendas. While many patients are simply lonely, cold or worried about other things, be on the look out for spouse abuse, child abuse or sexual abuse.

Abdominal Pain

Life threatening causes of abdominal pain include ectopic pregnancy, ruptured or dissecting aortic aneurysm, ruptured spleen, and MI. Consider these and thoracic etiologies (i.e pneumonia, PE) in every patient. Remember, however, that about 40% of patients will leave the ED without a diagnosis.

1. History: discern the location of maximal pain and if the pain is predominantly from obstruction/distention of an organ or peritoneal inflammation. Keep in mind that many obstructive disorders eventually lead to inflammation.
   Onset: abrupt vs. gradual.
   Timing: constant vs. intermittent.
   Character: crampy vs. sharp.
   Location: maximal pain, radiation.
   Vomiting: bilious or feculent.
   Diarrhea, constipation, urinary symptoms, urge to pass gas.
   Fever.
   PMH: Past episodes of similar pain. Cardiac, PUD, PVD, past operations, G#P#, LNMP, birth control, sexual history.

2. Physical: define the quadrant of maximal symptoms, and the character of the pain (i.e visceral or somatic).
   Vital signs.
   General appearance: patients with colicky pain tend to writhe, while those with peritoneal inflammation tend to lie still.
   Heart, lungs, and quick general examination.
   Abdomen: auscultate first, scars, light palpation, deeper palpation.
      Gentle percussion is equivalent to rebound tenderness.
      Note referred tenderness, cough tenderness. Hernias.
   Pelvic: mandatory in women. Cervical motion tenderness, adnexal tenderness, discharge, cultures.
   GU: penis, testicles mandatory.
   Rectal/Guaiac: tenderness (also mandatory).

3. Studies: confirm the diagnosis or narrow the differential.
   UA and pregnancy.
   CBC with differential.
   Electrolytes: indicated if vomiting or diuretic use.
   Glucose.
   LFTs, PT/PTT: in suspected liver/biliary disease.
   Amylase, Lipase, Ca^{++}: in suspected pancreatitis.
   Abdominal flat & upright with PA chest: to rule out free air, and to evaluate for SBO, ileus, constipation, or impaction; mildly helpful for stones.
   (Ileus is not a diagnosis. Look for the cause of an ileus).
   EKG: in older patients.

4. Initial Management: consider IVF, NGT and anti-emetics. Avoid ordering pain meds until the diagnosis is certain. Anti-emetics are not the treatment of SBO. See also Diarrhea/Nausea/Vomiting page 32.

Causes of Abdominal Pain

Does the patient fit into a typical syndrome for abdominal pain. Try to make the diagnosis early. Once the patient perforates and develops RLQ peritonitis, just about anyone can make the diagnosis. Typically, obstructed organs cause waves of crampy pain associated with vomiting, (e.g. SBO, biliary colic, kidney stones, and occasionally menstrual pain). Patients who lie still and flat, are quiet, or look toxic probably have peritonitis. Always exclude hernias. All bets are off if steroids are on board.

AAA disection: Pain radiating to back, may be associated with radicular findings, may have pulse findings, may have other stigmata of vascular disease, and in thinner individuals will feel the abdominal mass. Once the diagnosis is made, do not mash on the abdomen. Get the patient to surgery before he or she exsanguinates.

Cholelithiasis/Cholecystitis: Famous alliteration of Fat/Female/Fertile/Forty. May give history of fatty food intolerance. RUQ pain. Right shoulder pain.

PUD perforation: Sudden severe abdominal pain in patient who often has prior history of PUD. Patient has "board-like" abdomen with chemical peritonitis.

Mesenteric infarction: Pain out of proportion to exam. Patient is often older or has history of atrial fibrillation or aggressive atherosclerotic disease. The diagnosis must be made early. Later, when the patient develops peritonitis, the small intestine will be dead and the patient will follow.

Appendicitis: Usually has a prodrome of anorexia and central abdominal discomfort. Patient will refuse even their favorite food. May have nausea and vomiting. May have urge to "pass gas" to relieve pain. Early exam will be difficult with only minor RLQ pain. RLQ tenderness may be better appreciated on the rectal exam. Very difficult to distinguish at times from PID, except more GI sxs than PID. Serial exams and serial CBC may be helpful. Must be very suspicious in the young, the mentally impaired, and the old, when fever and RLQ pain is present.

Ectopic pregnancy: The patient is pregnant and has had some pain. Be suspicious of this diagnosis in any premenopausal female. The signs and symptoms are often lacking in this life-threatening disease.

Diverticulitis: LLQ pain in an older person. Mild peritoneal findings. Fever.

Gastroenteritis: Waves of crampy abdominal pain. The pain is relieved with diarrheal bowl movements. No peritonitis.

Mittelschmerz: LLQ or RLQ pain two weeks after the last menses. Paucity of GI sxs. Mild poritoneal tenderness.

PID: May have discharge and a prior history. Chandelier sign. Often admitted if sick. Tricky to separate from appendicitis.

SBO: Feculent vomiting without nausea in patient with prior abdominal surgery.

Renal colic: Waves of pain. Squirming about. Pain radiates to groin. Blood in urine.

Any pain that goes undiagnosed for more than six hours deserves a consult.

Acetaminophen Overdose

Acetaminophen poisoning causes only GI symptoms in the first 72 hours, therefore, changes in mental status cannot be due to acetaminophen.
If untreated, hepatic necrosis will eventually ensue and may lead to death.

History: exact amount and time of ingestion, was it an acetaminophen compound i.e. Tylenol#3 (codeine) or Tylenol PM (diphenhydramine)? Any other ingested material? Psychiatric history, prior ingestion, EtOH abuse, other medications, prior suicides.

Pathophysiology: Cytochrome P450 converts acetaminophen to N-acetyl-benzoqinoneimine (NAQ). This toxic metabolite is normally detoxified by conjugation with glutathione. In the presence of decreased glutathione stores (i.e. alcoholism) or consumption of stores as in overdose, NAQ binds covalently to hepatic macromolecules causing liver necrosis.

Management: ABC's, then:

1. Empty stomach with Ipecac or lavage if ingestion occurred within last 2-4 hours. In the ED gastric lavage is often favorable to Ipecac.

2. Activated charcoal is usually withheld, but may be alternated with mucomyst. Some toxicologists recommend using charcoal despite its possible competition with mucomyst absorption. If any drugs were co-ingested with acetaminophen, use charcoal if indicated.

3. Measure Acetaminophen level 4 hours post ingestion (levels drawn sooner may not reflect total GI absorption) and consult Rummack-Matthew nomogram to decide if to treat.

4. N-acetyl-cysteine (Mucomyst) 140mg/kg PO/NGT initially then, 70mg/kg q4h PO/NGT for 17 additional doses. Mucomyst is supplied as a 10% (10g/100ml) or 20% (20g/100ml) solution. Dilute with water, soda or juice 1:3 or 1:4 to make palatable.

5. Baseline CBC, SMA7, LFTs, PT, PTT, Tox screen.

6. Admit.

Acid-Base

1. Look at the pH. Is this patient acidemic or alkalemic?
2. Look at the pCO_2. Does the change in pCO_2 reflect the change in pH and thereby indicate a respiratory disorder, or does the change in pCO_2 reflect compensation for a primary metabolic disorder?

Metabolic Acidosis: respiratory compensation takes 12-24 hours to fully develop. Some relationships may be helpful:

1.2mmHg decrease In pCO_2 for every 1meq/l fall in HCO3

pCO_2=1.5[HCO3]+8

pCO_2 equals last two digits of pH.

Anion Gap (MUD PILES)
Methanol
Uremia
DKA
Paraldehyde,**P**henformin,**P**ropylene glycol
Iron, **INH**
Lactic acidosis
Ethanol, **E**thylene glycol
Salicylate, **S**tarvation

Non-anion Gap (HARD UP)
Hyperventilation (post)
Acetazolamide
Renal Tubular Acidosis
Diarrhea
Ureterosigmoidostomy
Pancreatic fistula

Metabolic Alkalosis: respiratory compensation unpredictable.
0.7mmHg rise in pCO_2 for every 1meq/l rise in HCO3.
pCO_2=0.9[HCO3]+9.

(D.VAGAL)
Diuretics
Vomiting
Aldosteronism
Gastric drainage
Alkali intake

Respiratory Acidosis: HCO3 usually does not rise above 32meq/l.
Acute: 1meq/l rise in HCO3 for every 10mmHg rise in pCO_2.
HCO3>32 suggests a superimposed metabolic alkalosis.
HCO3<22 suggests a superimposed metabolic acidosis.
Chronic: 3.5meq/l rise in HCO3 for every 10mmHG rise in pCO_2.

Respiratory Alkalosis: Adaptive fall in HCO3 occur in minutes.
Acute: 2meq/l fall in HCO3 for every 10 mmHg fall in pCO_2.
Chronic: 5meq/l fall in HCO3 for every 10 mmHg fall in PCO_2.

Alcohol

"The unhealthy conditions of city life are due to the crowding, the more uncertain means of livelihood, the greater influence of vice and alcoholism."
William T. Councilman, MD 1913.

Intoxication: patients demand thorough evaluation at the time of arrival and serial exams throughout their time in the ED. Waking patients every 30 minutes or so assures that they are not deteriorating neurologically (and suggests to them that your ED is not a good place to sleep it off).

History and physical:
- Look for evidence of trauma.
- Amount of EtOH, past history of seizures and DTs?
- Head: arousability, focal neurologic signs?
- Febrile: meningitis, aspiration, SBP?
- Abdomen: hepatitis, gastritis, PUD, pancreatitis?

Treatment:
1. Sedate if agitated.
   - Lorazepam 1-2mg IV/IM q5min until calm, then q2-4h.
   - Haloperidol 2-5mg q20min IV/IM until calm.
   - Clonidine for sympathetic symptoms.
2. Rule out infection if febrile.
3. Head CT if focal, agitated, head trauma, difficult to arouse.
4. IVF: D5 1/2NS + Thiamine100mg + Folate1mg + $MgSO_4$ 1gm + MVI amp
5. Thiamine before glucose.
6. Serial examinations while in ED.
7. Consider checking electrolytes, Mg^{++}.
8. Check pockets for medications. Consider checking phenytoin and phenobarbital levels.

Withdrawal: can occur within 8 hours of the last drink and before the BAL has returned to zero. Symptoms include tremor, insomnia, anxiety, nausea, vomiting, and diaphoresis. Hallucinations may occur, but the patients sensorium should otherwise be clear.

Seizures: may begin between 8 and 24 hours after the last drink and before the BAL has returned to zero. They generally occur before onset of DTs. Withdrawal cannot be assumed responsible for seizures that begin after the onset of delirium, are focal or multiple, or occur in febrile or traumatized patients.

DTs: are rare in patients less than 30, and usually occur 48hrs to 14 days after the last drink. Manifestations include confusion, hyperactivity, HTN, tachycardia, fever, diaphoresis, and volume depletion.

Wernicke's Encephalopathy: consists of the classic triad of cognitive impairment, ocular dysfunction, and ataxia.

Allergic Reactions

"A man cannot have better fortune than to be able, nor a better temper than be willing, to save many." Cicero.

Allergic reactions represent a continuum of disorders from simple cutaneous urticaria to anaphylaxis. Quick initial assessment is mandatory as rapid treatment can be lifesaving. Management is based on signs and symptoms at presentation and during a reasonable period of observation.

ABCs: then, depending on severity, any or all of the following:

Oxygen by NC of FM
Epinephrine 0.3-0.5cc SQ (1:1,000)
3-5 cc IV (1:10,000)
IV access 1 or 2 large bore IVs then NS or LR
Diphenhydramine 50mg PO/IV
Cimetidine 300mg PO/IV
Methylprednisolone 125mg IV or Prednisone 40mg PO

Airway: examine for laryngeal stridor and angioedema. Get help if either is apparent.

Breathing: assess rate, depth, ease of respirations. Auscultate for wheezes. If it is difficult to discern between wheezing and laryngeal stridor treat as if airway closure is imminent. A peak flow may be useful.

Circulation: Blood pressure, peripheral cyanosis, shock. Hypotensive patients should receive 2-4L of LR or NS rapidly.

Anaphylaxis: requires SQ or IV epinephrine and aggressive fluid resuscitation as well as all adjunctive measures. Admission for observation is usually indicated.

Wheezes/Angioedema/Laryngeal stridor: require treatment with Oxygen, epinephrine IV or SQ, nebs, IV access and adjunctive therapy with IV Diphenhydramine, Cimetidine, and steroids. At least six hours of observation is indicated.

Cutaneous Urticaria: (Hives) may be treated conservatively with PO or IM Benadryl and PO Cimetidine. Additionally, SQ epinephrine may speed resolution of symptoms and is relatively safe in patients without cardiovascular disease. Steroids take 6-12 hours to take effect, but a PO/IV bolus followed by a three day pulse may prevent return of symptoms.

Asthma

The goal of therapy is to relieve airflow obstruction while maintaining oxygenation. Therapy and disposition in adults are based on peak flows to document improvement or decline.

Before the History and Physical:

1. O_2 at 2-4 L/min by nasal canulae in adults or mask in kids.
2. Albuterol nebs - unit dose (2.5mg or 0.5cc of a 0.5% solution diluted in 3cc NS) q15-20minutes times three.
   (0.15mg/kg/dose up to 2.5mg in kids).
3. Pulse Ox-if less than 90% get help.
4. Peak Flow measurement-if less than 100 in adults get help.
5. ABG if patient looks bad-PCO_2>40 bad sign.

History and Physical:

Time, onset, severity of symptoms of present exacerbation.
Current meds and last use of each, recent use of steroids.
Prior hospitalizations, prior intubations, steroid use, heart disease.
Vital signs especially respiratory rate, level of distress, level of consciousness, use of accessory muscles. (The sickest patients are usually bolt upright and diaphoretic unless they are supine and coding).
Auscultation. The sickest patients often move so little air the chest is silent.
Pulsus paradoxus is a bad sign.

Further Management:

6. Methylprednisolone 125mg IV (2mg/kg in children) in patients without improvement after 1 or 2 nebs, or patients currently taking steroids.
7. Theophylline level.
8. Reevaluate patient after first neb and third neb:
   Perform peak-flow, auscultate chest, talk to patient.
9. CXR in patients with cough with sputum, asymmetric breath sounds, or admitted.
10. CBC if febrile, draw before steroids administered.

Disposition:

Good response: no SOB or wheezes, PF > 300.
    Observe of 1 hour after last neb, then d/c to home on inhaled beta-agonist and steroid taper if steroids given in ED. Follow up with PMD in 1-3 days.
Poor response: no improvement or patient in ED for >4 hours.
    Admit to ICU or medical bed as appropriate.
Intermediate response: feeling better but improved only marginally.
    Hit with steroids if not already, consider theophylline, and reevaluate after another three nebs.

Asthma (continued)

Other Modalities:

Subcutaneous Beta-agonist
Epinephrine 0.3mg 1:1000 SQ q20min up to 3 doses.
(0.01mg/kg up to 0.3mg in children).
Terbutaline 0.25mg (0.1%) SQ q2-6hrs prn.
(0.01mg/kg up to 0.25mg in children).

Theophylline
6mg/kg IV bolus if level 0, then 0.6mg/kg/hr continuous
If level known but not zero, bolus 0.5mg/kg for every 1.0ug/ml bump in level desired.
Monitor levels to adjust thereafter.

Magnesium Sulfate: the new trend in therapy.
1gm in 100ccD5W over 20 minutes. Repeat once prn.

Ipratropium Bromide (Atrovent)
MDI or neb (when available) alternating with beta-agonist.

Atropine Nebs
Used as an adjunct in both adults and children.

Mechanical ventilation
Indications: ventilatory failure, or impending failure, poor MS, hypercapnia, hypoxia.
Initial Settings: AC or IMV, Rate=14, Vt=10ml/kg, I:E 1:3, no peep. Watch peak pressures as barotrauma is the major complication. ABG in 15-20 minutes.
Get patient upstairs.

Death due to asthma is on the rise; be aggressive.

Back Pain

"I have often allayed the patients anxiety by reassuring myself that I shall never see them again." Anonymous.

History: always consider abdominal aortic aneurysm, pancreatitis, kidney stone, PID, pyelonephritis, and other "non-back" causes of pain. Consider trauma and occupational history.

Physical: feel for AAA, attempt to differentiate between radicular and non-radicular symptoms. Strait leg raises should illicit pain below the knee to suggest radiculopathy.

Treat pain in the department with parenteral NSAIDs or PO/IM narcotics after initial evaluation. (Good public relations).

LS Spine X-rays: are over ordered by most physicians.

- Relative indications:
  - extremes of age
  - history of CA
  - workman's compensation
  - trauma
  - long-standing pain

Treatment/Disposition

Lumbosacral strain: based on the degree of injury and severity of symptoms.

1. Complete bed-rest for two days using high dose NSAIDs plus muscle relaxants or oral narcotics:
   Ibuprofen 600mg PO q6h for 2 days then prn plus
   Cyclobenzaprine 10mg PO tid for 2 days or
   Tylenol with codeine i-ii PO q4-6h for 2 days or
   Diazepam 5mg PO Q6H prn.
2. Gradual return to normal activity over 2-4 weeks.
3. Two days off then one week light duty.
4. F/U with primary care physician within one week.

Suspected disk disease: follow up sooner with orthopedic/neurosurgical referral if no primary care follow up exists.

Objective nerve root signs, unstable fractures, intractable pain: ED consultation with orthopedics or neurosurgery for possible admission.

Burns

Burns are classified by severity based on degree, percent body surface area (BSA), region involved, and mechanism of injury. Initial management is based on burn severity, with attention paid to ABCs, evaluation for inhalation injury, protection of burns from contamination, initial fluid resuscitation, tetanus prophylaxis, and adequate analgesia.

The degree of burn may be difficult to assess but is based on the amounts of epidermis and dermis involved.

1° burns are erythematous, painful and mildly edematous.
2° burns affect the dermis and commonly blister.
3° burns involve the entire dermis & do not heal spontaneously.

Percent BSA is approximated in adults by the rule of nines: head and each arm-9%, leg and front or back of torso-18%, perineum-1%. The head is relatively larger in children.

The American Burn Association categorizes burns as follows:
Major burn: >25% BSA; functionally significant involvement of hands, feet, face, perineum; electrical, inhalational, or other concomitant injury; severe pre-existing medical problems.
Moderate burn: 15-25% BSA; uncomplicated involvement of the hands, feet, face, perineum.
Minor Burn: <15% BSA.

Management

1. Airway: evaluate for inhalational injury: facial burns, singed nose hair, sooty sputum, carbonized snot. Stabilize C-spine prn.

2. Breathing: Auscultate. CXR/ABG/COHb if inhalation suspected.

3. Circulation: 1-2 large bore IVs. Fluid resuscitation is guided by the Parkland Formula: 4ml/kg/%BSA of LR: 1/2 given over the first 8 hours, 1/2 given over the remaining 16 hours. Foley.

4. Administer tetanus.

5. Minor 1st and 2nd degree burns are soothed well with application of gauze soaked in cold sterile saline. More extensive burns can cause hypothermia and cool applications should not be given. Cleanse all burns with mild soap or bacteriostatic solution and debride all nonviable tissue. Remove blister fluid. Apply layer of silver sulfadiazine and apply dry sterile cotton gauze dressing.

6. Narcotic analgesia prn.

7. All moderate and major burns generally get admitted. Consider transfer to a burn unit.

8. Minor burns may be discharged to plastic surgery or primary care follow-up depending on severity. Have patient follow up for a 24 hour wound check unless extremely minor.

Cardiac Arrest

VF and pulseless VT

ABCs
Initiate CPR[1]
Attach defibrillator/monitor

Defibrillate at 200J
Defibrillate at 300J
Defibrillate at 360J

Continue CPR
Intubate
IV Access[2]

Epinephrine 1mg IVP[3]
Defibrillate 360J
Lidocaine 1.5mg/kg IVP[4]
Defibrillate 360J
Bretylium 5mg/kg IVP[5]
Defibrillate 360J

Consider Magnesium, Procainamide, and sodium bicarbonate
Continue medications and shocks in alternating fashion

[1]Precordial thump is acceptable if witnessed arrest, no pulse, and no defibrillator available.
[2]Peripheral vein: antecubital or external jugular.
[3]Repeat Q3-5min. Consider escalating doses.
[4]Repeat Q3-5min up to 3mg/kg.
[5]Repeat Bretylium 10mg/kg in 5 min.

Guidelines on this page and pages 22-24 adapted from:
Emergency Cardiac Care Committee and Subcommittees, American Heart Association. Guidlines for cardiolpulmonary resusciation and emergency cardiac care. III: Adult ACLS. JAMA. 1992; 268: 2199-2250.

Cardiac Arrest (continued)

Pulseless Electrical Activity

ABCs
Initiate CPR
Intubate
IV Access

Assess blood flow using Doppler ultrasound

Consider possible causes:
Hypovolemia, Hypoxia, Cardiac Tamponade
Tension Pneumothorax, Hypothermia, PE, Overdose
Hyperkalemia[1], Acidosis[2], MI

Epinephrine 1mg IVP[3]
Atropine 1mg IVP[4]

Asystole

ABCs
Initiate CPR
Intubate
IV Access

Confirm Asystole in more than one lead

Consider possible causes:
Hypoxia, Hyperkalemia[1], Hypokalemia
Preexisting acidosis[2], Drug overdose[2], Hypothermia

Consider transcutaneous pacing[5]

Epinephrine 1mg IVP[3]

Atropine 1mg IVP[4]

[1]Administer Sodium Bicarbonate 1meq/kg
[2]Consider Bicarbonate for known bicarbonate-responsive acidosis, tricyclic overdose, or if intubated and long arrest interval.
[3]Repeat Q3-5min. Consider escalating doses.
[4]Repeat Q3-5min up to 0.04mg/kg IV. Consider shorter dosing interval.
[5]Possibly helpful if performed early and simultaneously with drugs.

Cardiac Arrhythmias

Bradycardia

ABC's
Vitals
IV Access, Oxygen
Cardiac monitor, Pulse oximeter, BP cuff.
↓
Serious signs or symptoms[1]

Yes
↓
Atropine 0.5-1.0mg IVP[2]
↓
Trans-cutaneous Pacer
↓
Dopamine 5-20ug/kg/min IV
↓
Epinephrine 2-10ug/min IV
↓
Isoproterenol[4]

No
↓
Mobitz II or Third Degree[3] HB?

- Yes → Apply Trans-cutaneous Pacer → Trans-venous pacer
- No → Observation

[1]Chest pain, SOB, decreased consciousness, hypotension, shock, CHF, MI.
[2]Repeat Q3-5min up to 0.04mg/kg. Consider shorter intervals. Use with caution in patients with Mobitz II and complete HB with wide QRS.
[3]Never treat 3rd degree HB with ventricular escape beats with lidocaine.
[4]Use with extreme caution at low doses.

Tachycardia

Unstable or Serious Signs or Symptoms

If ventricular rate > 150 beats/min, prepare for immediate cardioversion
May give brief trial of medications based on specific arrhythmias
Check O_2 saturation and IV access
Ready intubation equipment and suction
Premedicate if possible
Synchronized cardioversion

Atrial flutter/PSVT	Atrial fibrillation	VT
50J	100J	100J
100J	200J	200J
200J	300J	300J
300J	360J	360J
360J		

Cardiac Arrhythmias (continued)

Ventricular Tachycardia (VT) - Stable

Lidocaine 1-1.5mg/kg IVP
↓
Lidocaine 0.5-0.75mg/kg IV q5-10 minutes up to 3mg/kg
↓
Procainamide 20-30mg/min IV up to 17mg/kg total dose
↓
Bretylium 5-10mg/kg IV over 8-10 min up to 30mg/kg
↓
Synchronized cardioversion

Wide Complex Tachycardia - Stable

Lidocaine 1-1.5mg/kg IVP
↓
Lidocaine 0.5-0.75mg/kg IV q5-10 minutes up to 3mg/kg
↓
Adenosine 6mg rapid IVP
↓
Adenosine 12mg rapid IVP
↓
Adenosine 12mg rapid IVP
↓
Procainamide 20-30mg/min IV up to 17mg/kg total dose
↓
Bretylium 5-10mg/kg IV over 8-10 min up to 30mg/kg
↓
Synchronized cardioversion

PSVT

Vagal maneuvers
Adenosine 6mg rapid IVP
Adenosine 12mg rapid IVP
Adenosine 12mg rapid IVP
QRS Complex width?

Narrow and BP Stable	Wide (presume VT)
Verapamil 2.5-5mg IV	Lidocaine 1-1.5mg/kg
↓	Procainamide 20-30mg/min up to 17mg/kg total dose
Verapamil 5-10 mg IV	Synchronized cardioversion
↓	
Consider: Digoxin, Diltiazem, Beta-blockers	
↓	
Synchronized cardioversion	

Atrial Fibrillation or Flutter

Diltiazem 0.25mg/kg IVP over 2 minutes.
If no result, wait 15 min and administer 0.35mg/kg IVP over 2 minutes.
If still no result, consider beta-blocker, verapamil, digoxin, procainamide, or quinidine. *Use caution with multiple agents.*
Consider anticoagulation for all longstanding cases of atrial fibrillation.

Chest Pain

Assume every patient is having myocardial ischemia until proven otherwise.
Patients should receive O_2 by nasal canulae, a full set of vitals, cardiac monitoring, and be disrobed to the waist.

History: attempt to qualify pain as cardiac or non-cardiac in origin, then if non-cardiac to rule out any life threatening cause.

HPI: *OPQRST*

Onset: when did it start, activity at the time.
Provocative/palliative factors: what makes it start/stop.
Quality: sharp, dull, burning, boring, knifelike, squeezing.
Radiation: arms, jaw, tingling, paresthesia.
Severity: generally 1 to 10 with ten most severe.
Timing: early morning, constant, intermittent.
Associated symptoms: diaphoresis, nausea, vomiting.

PMH: past cardiac history, PVD, medications, coexisting disease, cardiac risk factors.

Physical: is pain reproducible by palpation? Murmurs, wheezes, crackles, consolidation, pleural rub.

Chest X-ray: rule out pneumonia and pneumothorax and evaluate cardiac silhouette, widened mediastinum, mass or rib fracture.

EKG: Old EKG for comparison is essential.

Identify strengths of patients story and evaluate EKG for ischemia:

1. Good story with EKG changes: the diagnosis will be either acute MI (still having pain) or unstable angina (now pain free). Pain-free patients should receive ASA and consideration of heparin. See Myocardial Infarction page 55.

2. Bad story with EKG changes: will need to be evaluated for why their EKG changed. An attending will need to decide if an early catheterization is warranted. Patients should probably go to the CCU, although they may be managed in the step-down unit if their cardiologist is comfortable with that.

3. Good story, no EKG changes: perhaps the toughest. Here age and cardiac risk factors come into play, although even young patients without risk factors should be taken seriously. A cardiologist or the patient's private attending should be called and probably will admit.

4. Bad story, no EKG changes: often admitted as r/o MI to go home the next morning and follow up with PMD. Provide follow up and document specific instructions to return if pain changes in any way etc. Think about PE.

Chest Pain (continued)

Once myocardial ischemia is ruled out, concentrate on the other life threatening causes for chest pain. Consider PE and aortic aneurysm in every patient.

Differential Diagnosis

Ischemia
- Myocardial infarction
- Unstable angina
- Variant/Prinzmetal's angina
- Stable angina
- Aortic stenosis

Other Cardiovascular
- Aortic Dissection/Aneurysm
- Pericarditis
- Myocarditis
- Hypertrophic cardiomyopathy
- IHSS
- Mitral valve prolapse
- Cardiac tumor

Pulmonary/Mediastinal
- Pulmonary embolism
- Mediastinitis
- Mediastinal emphysema
- Pneumothorax
- Pneumonia
- Pleurisy
- Pulmonary infarction
- Mediastinal mass
- Tracheitis

Musculoskeletal
- Costochondritis
- Precordial catch
- Rib fracture
- Pectoralis major/minor pain
- Xiphisternal arthritis
- Cervical/Thoracic disc

Other
- Herpes Zoster (Shingles)
- Hyperventilation
- Thoracic outlet syndrome
- Chest wall thrombophlebitis

Gastrointestinal
- Esophagitis/Esophageal spasm
- PUD
- Biliary disease
- Pancreatitis

Psychiatric
- Panic disorder
- Somatization disorder
- NOS

Disposition: In the absence of a definitive diagnosis, rule out life threatening causes and establish adequate follow-up before sending the patient home.

CHF/Pulmonary Edema

CHF and pulmonary edema present acutely, with or without history of prior cardiovascular disease, or sub-acutely, with history of previous episodes of CHF or CVD. Pulmonary edema may also result from non-cardiac causes such as ARDS or decreased oncotic forces.

Initial Evaluation: assess ABCs and mentation and provide:

1. Oxygen-by NC or FM depending on severity.
2. Cardiac monitor.
3. Vitals.
4. Pulse-ox, CBC, SMA-7, Digoxin level. ABG?
5. Call for stat EKG, PCXR.

History (brief): onset, prior episodes, CP, DOE, PND, orthopnea, meds, history of prior cardiac disease, non-compliance, dietary indiscretion. Palpitations may suggest SVT with impaired diastolic filling as a cause.

Physical (more brief): cyanosis, tachypnea, neck veins, crackles (rales), S3, murmurs, rubs, or muffled heart sounds, peripheral edema.

Initial Management: is aimed at decreasing preload and treating symptoms. *If signs, symptoms or history of AS, IHSS or MS exist, get help - these patients can bottom out with intervention.*

6. Nitrates: venodilators that act to redistribute preload to the periphery.
   Keep SBP > 100-110.
   NTG 0.4mg SL Q5-10min PRN times 3. (Nice bolus)
   NTP 1/2" to 2" applied to chest. (Less aggressive)
   NTG drip (100mg/500ccD5W) begin at 5ug/min.

7. MSO4: decreases anxiety/dyspnea, promotes venodilation.
   MSO4 1-2mg IV Q10min PRN.

8. Diuretics-remove excess volume.
   Furosemide 20-40mg IV in patients without CRF or prior use.
   Furosemide 40-100mg IV if on chronic therapy or CRI.
   Patients with oliguric renal failure will need dialysis.

Interventions/Studies: Patients with or without prior CV history and acute onset of symptoms have suffered an acute derangement. Work-up is essential for proper and rapid therapy of the underlying cause. Consider:
ECHO: to rule out effusion, tamponade, valvular abnormality, or hypocontractility.
PA Catheter: guides therapy and evaluates PA pressure.
V/Q scan: consider PE.

COPD

"Tobacco is the second of the socially acceptable drugs." Mack Lipkin, MD.

Search for the cause of the acute exacerbation and tailor therapy to the severity of the disease. Always treat hypoxemia, but remember that oxygen may abolish the patient's respiratory drive.

1. Initial assessment: Cardiac monitor, pulse-ox, draw bloods.
Look for signs of respiratory failure: poor mental status, central cyanosis, abnormal vital signs, inadequate rate or depth of respiration?

2. O2 at 1-3L via NC, or sufficient to raise O2 sat to 85-90% (PaO2 50-60mmHg). Treatment of hypoxia is paramount. Once pO2 is in adequate range, treatment of hypercarbia is mechanical ventilation.

3. Albuterol nebs (unit dose) q30min times three.

4. History/Physical/Labs: severity and etiology of exacerbation.
Onset and duration of symptoms: increased cough, sputum, fever, pleuritic CP. Recent trips to ED, hospitalizations, steroid use. Meds with dosages. Co-existing disease. Tachypnea, tachycardia, fever, accessory muscles, breath sounds, clubbing, cyanosis.
ABG after about 20-30 minutes of O2.
CBC, Theophylline level.
CXR to rule out PTX from ruptured bleb or infiltrate.
Peak flow may aid in deciding on disposition.

6. Theophylline may be helpful in patients who take it orally, but is of controversial benefit. Bolus 1mg/kg IV over 30 minutes for every 2mg/L bump in level desired, continue at 0.6mg/kg/hr continuous IV infusion if admitted.

7. Ipratropium bromide is of proven benefit in COPD and may help during acute exacerbation. 4 puffs to start then 4 puffs alternating with nebs.

8. Methylprednisolone 1-2mg/kg IV or PO equivalent.

9. Disposition: mild cases may be treated with O2, nebs, PO steroids, theophylline, and discharged on PO antibiotics, MDIs and steroid taper. More severe cases will need to be admitted. Counsel all smokers to stop smoking. Ask patient if service connected.

Coma and Disordered Consciousness

1. Stabilization:
   Airway/C-spine immobilization: nasal airway (semi-comatose) or oral airway (comatose) as needed.
   Breathing: O_2, check rate and depth of respiration.
   Circulation: assess BP/P, establish IV access and apply cardiac monitor.
   EKG.
   D50%-50ml+Naloxone 2mg+Thiamine 100mg IV. Consider flumazenil.
   Temperature.
2. Clinical Assessment:
   A. Level of responsiveness: sleep, lethargy, stupor, coma.
      AVPU-Alert, Voice, Pain, Unresponsive.
      Glasgow Coma Scale GCS (3-15)

Eye opening (E)	
Spontaneous	4
To Loud Voice	3
To Pain	2
Nil	1
Motor Response (M)	
Obeys Verbal Command	6
Localizes Pain	5
Flexion Withdrawal	4
Decorticate rigidity	3
Decerebrate rigidity	2
Nil	1
Verbal Response (V)	
Oriented/converses	5
Disoriented/converses	4
Inappropriate words	3
Incomprehensible	2
Nil	1

   B. Brainstem Signs:
      Decortication: flexion of wrists and elbows and supination of arms suggests bilateral damage in the hemispheres.
      Decerebration:extension of wrists and elbows with arm pronation suggests damage to midbrain or diencephalon.
   C. Pupils:
      Equal and Reactive: suggests an intact midbrain.
      Unilateral large: ipsilateral midbrain lesion or compression from herniation.
      Bilateral large: severe midbrain damage or herniation or sympathomimetic or anticholinergic toxin.
      Bilateral small: metabolic encephalopathy, narcotic OD, bilateral hemispherical lesion or bilateral pons damage.
   D. Caloric Stimulation: cold water in ear.
      Tonic deviation of both eyes towards stimulus implies intact brainstem.
      Fast nystagmus away from tonic deviation suggests an intact opposite cerebral hemisphere.

Coma (continued)

3. Studies/Laboratory:
   CBC, Electrolytes, BUN, Creatinine, Glucose, $NH4^{+}$, Ca^{++}, Osm.
   Serum or urine Tox Screen.
   Pulse-ox, ABG, HbCO.
   CT Scan of Head (non-contrast): does not rule out an anatomic lesion.
   LP: meningitis, encephalitis.

4. Etiologies: coma is caused by either bilateral hemispherical damage or suppression by drugs or toxins, or brainstem lesion or metabolic derangement that damages or suppresses the RAS.

CT scan usually negative
- Drugs or Toxins: EtOH, opiates, benzodiazepines, anticholinergics, etc.
- Metabolic encephalopathy: hypoxia, hypercarbia, DKA, HONC, hypoglycemia, uremia, hepatic encephalopathy, hyponatremia, hypocalcemia, CO, hypothermia, malignant hyperthermia, thyroid dysfunction, hypoadrenalism, fever, sepsis.
- Meningitis/encephalitis: bacterial, viral, HIV related, TTP.
- Seizure disorder: sub-clinical seizure vs. post-ictal state.
- Hypertensive encephalopathy.
- Wernicke's encephalopathy.

CT scan usually positive
- Head trauma: contusion, edema.
- Intracerebral hemorrhage: epidural hematoma, subdural hematoma, bilateral SAH, basal ganglia, thalamic, cerebellar, pontine or midbrain hemorrhage.
- Cerebrovascular accident (CVA) - may be negative in first 24 hours.
- Intracerebral mass: abscess, tumor.
- Basilar artery thrombosis.
- Hydrocephalus

CVA

Stroke causes sudden disruption of cerebral perfusion along a particular territory.
It presents most often as a focal neurological deficit, but may also present as depressed level of consciousness, headache, dizziness, ataxia, vertigo, facial weakness, aphasia or visual loss.

Address ABCs, stabilize the patient, and order HCT to define whether the stroke is due to sudden occlusion of a vessel by thrombus or embolus, (ischemic stroke) or bleeding, (hemorrhagic stroke).

1. ABCs: check airway reflexes and insert the proper airway. Consider C-spine injury. Assess depth and rate of respiration, and check for abnormal patterns of respiration. Check BP, pulse, and distal perfusion.

2. Start O_2 (O_2 is becoming controversal, follow local practice)., cardiac monitor, pulse-ox, IV NS at KVO, draw bloods. Avoid dextrose, hypotonic, or large amounts of fluids unless hypotensive.

3. History: prior CVA, cardiac arrhythmias, HTN, drug use, medications.

4. Physical: head trauma, C-spine, neck stiffness, murmur, bruits, disks. Level of consciousness, GCS, pupils, CNs, cerebellar exam, muscles strength, sensory loss.

5. Studies:
   - Labs: CBC, SMA6, glucose, PT,PTT.
   - EKG: arrhythmia, thrombus.
   - C-spine: rule out fracture.
   - PCXR: rule out aspiration, evaluate cardiac size.

6. Head CT without contrast: rule out hemorrhage.

7. Complications:
   - Seizures: diazepam initially then load with dilantin.
   - HTN: consider treatment with short acting agents. Patients may need the increased perfusion pressures.
   - Increased ICP: hyperventilation, mannitol, steroids.
   - Glucose: you may want to avoid both hypoglycemia and hyperglycemia.

8. Consult neurology for ischemic stroke, neurosurgery for hemorrhagic.

Diarrhea, Nausea and Vomiting

Consider IVF repletion and symptomatic relief early.

1. History: concentrate on severity of symptoms, and explore etiologies.
   - Onset: acute vs. chronic, duration, severity.
   - Number of vomiting episodes or BMs per day or per hour.
   - Character of emesis: clear, bile, blood, feculent.
   - Watery, loose, poorly formed or simply frequent formed BMs.
   - Appearance of stool: blood, floating, (unusually) malodorous.
   - Past medical history: arthritis, bowel surgery, pancreatitis, AIDS.
   - Travel, EtOH abuse.
   - Meds: laxatives, antacids, antibiotics, use of antidiarrheals.
   - Fever.

2. Physical: concentrate on degree of hypovolemia and coexisting disease.
   - Orthostatic vital signs, Temperature.
   - General level of nutrition.
   - Rectal, Guaiac, and examination of stool.
   - Abdominal exam: mass, tenderness, peritoneal signs.

3. Labs: CBC, SMA7, AST, ALT, Alk phos, Bili, Amylase.
   - Stool studies for diarrhea:
     - Acute Diarrhea: Wright Stain for fecal WBCs.
     - Bloody Diarrhea: Culture for Salmonella, Shigella, Campylobacter.
     - Travel or HIV+: Ova and Parasites.
     - Antibiotic use: C-difficile.
     - Seafood: Vibrio.
   - X-ray: acute abdominal series (flat and upright with PA chest).
     - Rule out ileus/SBO, free air, kidney stone.

4. Therapy: Treat symptoms of hypovolemia and nausea or vomiting. Nausea and vomiting secondary to ileus or SBO is best treated with an NGT. Avoid treating acute diarrhea as it is most often viral and self limited. Normal saline volume repletion makes patients feel better. Young patients can tolerate one or two liters of fluid give very quickly.

Anti-emetics:
- Promethazine (Phenergan) 12.5mg IV or 25mg IM.
- Prochlorperazine (Compazine) 5mg slow IV or 10mg IM (watch for dystonic rxn).

Anti-cholinergic: helpful for spasm.
- Dicyclomine (Bentyl) 20mg IM.
- Glycopyrrolate (Robinul) 0.1-0.2mg IV.

Antidiarrheals: only non-inflammatory conditions.
- Bismuth (Pepto-Bismol) 2 tabs or 30ml PO Q30min PRN.
- Loperamide (Imodium) 4mg PO then 2mg PO q unformed stool.

Antibiotics: if non-salmonella bacterial enteritis suspected.
- Ciprofloxacin 500mg BID in adults only.

DKA/HONC

Patients with DKA and HONC present with varying levels of ECF depletion, glucose elevation, and acidosis. ED management should concentrate on ABCs and initial volume resuscitation.

The goal of therapy is resolution of the acidosis, not a normal glucose.

Evaluation: concentrate on what precipitated the problem.

History: inquire specifically about noncompliance, coexisting illness, fever, chest pain, medications and PMH.

Physical: assess volume status, BP, pulse, orthostatics, temperature.

Labs/Studies: CBC, SMA7, UA, Serum Ketones, Amylase, EKG, beta hCG. An ABG usually is only necessary for morning report.

Management:

1. Bolus normal saline to restore BP to normal range, then give 2-3 liters over the first 2-3 hours to restore ECF losses. DKA patients are commonly 4 to 8 liters depleted while HONC patients may be over 10 liters behind. Once the patient is euvolemic, 1/2 normal saline is used to replace free water. If an acidosis still exists when the glucose reaches 300, add D5 or D10 to the IVF as needed.

2. Regular Insulin 0.1-0.15 units/kg/hr for DKA and 0.05 U/kg/hr in HONC. Use continuous IV infusion and avoid boluses; a precipitous fall in glucose can cause cerebral edema and hypokalemia. Dilute 50U Insulin in 100ccNS (0.5U/cc).

3. KCl is usually necessary as DKA and HONC patients are usually total body potassium depleted, by because of the acidosis, serum K^+ is usually high initially. Add KCl to IVF at 15-20meq/hr when K^+ drops below 4.

4. Bicarbonate is rarely indicated unless the pH is less than 6.9 or the patient exhibits cardiac arrhythmias. Place one or two amps in the IVF bag and avoid boluses.

5. Check finger-stick Q1H and SMA-7 Q4H while in ED.

Ear

Otitis Media: occurs most commonly in children with prior URI. Organisms include S.Pneumoniae 30%, H.Influenza 20%, M.Catarrhalis 10-20%, S.Pyogenes 2-3%, S.Aureus 1-2%, E.Coli, and Klebsiella. Group B strep can occur in first 6 wks of life.

Symptoms: ear pain, pulling at ears, and fever are most common. Babies often cry when laid flat.

Signs: examine color, position, transparency and mobility of the TM. Erythema and bulging of TM are common. Decreased motion of the TM on pneumatic otoscopy is the most sensitive indicator of disease. Exclude mastoiditis.

Rx: Amoxicillin 40mg/kg/day PO divided tid is the drug of choice. Beta-lactimase producing strains of H.flu and M.Cat are on the rise. If antibiotics have recently been used or child has a history of amoxicillin resistance: Cefaclor 40mg/kg/day PO divided tid or, Amoxicillin/Clavulanate 40mg/kg/day PO divided tid can be initiated.

Otitis Externa: is an infection of the pinnae and canal. Local trauma or the presence of water in the canal (i.e. swimmer's ear) are common causes. Pain can be excruciating and swelling severe enough to completely occlude the ear canal and make examination difficult.

Rx: If the ear canal is completely occluded a small wick must be inserted to keep the canal open and allow topical antibiotics to penetrate deeper structures. If a wick cannot be inserted, ENT should be consulted in the ED. Topical antibacterial/ corticosteroid preparations are the mainstay of treatment.
Cortisporin Otic Solution 4 ggts q6hrs for 10 days. Oral antibiotics with staphylococcal coverage (i.e. cephalexin) may be used if infection is severe.

Diabetic or otherwise immune compromised patients are at high risk for developing a severe Pseudomonas infection known as malignant otitis and should receive PO antibiotics and urgent ENT follow up if infection is mild and ENT consult for admission and IV antibiotics if infection is severe.

Ectopic Pregnancy

Ectopic pregnancy kills young women. Consider it in every woman with a positive pregnancy test and vaginal bleeding or abdominal pain.

Risk Factors: history of prior ectopic pregnancy, history of PID, infertility, tubal ligation, IUD, recent elective abortion.

History: $G_{\#}P_{fpal}$, abdominal pain: onset, severity, quality; vaginal bleeding:onset and amount; history of sexually transmitted diseases, LNMP.

Physical: vital signs and orthostatics, abdominal tenderness, peritoneal signs, pelvic: adnexal tenderness or fullness.

Labs: CBC, Type and Screen, Rh factor, Quantitative beta-hCG.

Sonography: used to assess whether a gestational sac exists.
- Transabdominal: gestational sac at 5-6 weeks.
- Transvaginal: gestational sac at 4-5 weeks. (Beta >1500).

Culdocentesis: non-clotting blood is proof of blood in peritoneal cavity, but a negative aspirate proves nothing.

Management:

1. ABCs. Assess hemodynamic status.
2. 2 large bore IVs with NS or LR infusion if hypotensive.
3. CBC, T&S or T&C, Quantitative Beta-hCG.
4. Consult OB/GYN.
5. Sonogram if stable, culdocentesis if resuscitation given, to OR if unstable.

Elbow

The elbow is a hinge joint consisting of three articulations within a single capsule. Acute injuries occur from falls or from direct impact. Bony injury is more common than ligamentous. A number of soft tissue conditions may present as well.

History: document mechanism and time of injury, past injuries to elbow, history of arthritis or other conditions, and the use of ice, immobilization and meds.

Physical: inspect and document distal pulses and condition of overlying skin. Observe for deformity. Palpate both epicondyles, the radial head, and olecranon. Test integrity of median, ulnar and radial nerves.

Consider early and liberal use of pain medications, an IV if dislocation is confirmed, and bloods and pre-op labs if going to the OR.

Radiology: (standard views)

AP with elbow in neutral position.

AP with elbow in supination.

Lateral with elbow at 90° : Look for either an anterior or posterior fat pad sign. Either implies a joint effusion, but only the posterior fat pad sign is 100% specific for an intra-articular fracture.

Fractures

Proximal radius fractures may be associated with fractures or dislocations of the proximal or distal radioulnar joints. Simple non-displaced fractures may be placed in a sling or posterior splint with RICE and orthopedic follow up in one week. Displaced or angulated fractures must be followed up sooner and comminuted (Neer fractures) or severely displaced or angulated fractures should receive an ortho consult in the ED. Olecranon fractures occur from falls or direct blows and may be associated with ulnar nerve palsy, radial head dislocation (Monteggia fracture) or olecranon dislocation. Simple non-displaced olecranon fractures are placed in a posterior splint with liberal ortho follow up. More complex injuries require ED orthopedic consultation. Distal humerus fractures may affect one or both condyles and are often associated with ulnar nerve damage and compartment syndrome. Get orthopedics involved early.

Soft Tissue Problems

Epicondylitis: (Tennis elbow) is an overuse disorder characterized by pain just distal to the lateral epicondyle. Rx: NSAIDs, immobilization and follow-up.

Olecranon bursitis: causes warmth swelling and pain over the apex of the elbow. It may be traumatic, inflammatory or septic, and diagnosis is made by aspiration under sterile conditions and fluid analysis.

Epistaxis

Calm the patient. Tackle the nosebleed first and save the history for when hemorrhage is under control.

Most bleeds are anterior, from Kesselbach's plexus on the nasal septum. Other sites include the turbinates and posterior sites. Bleeding from both nares suggests a posterior source.

Many EDs carry inflatable balloons for temporary control of both anterior and posterior bleeds.

1. Gown both you and the patient. Wear gloves and eye-wear.

2. Even if the bleeding has stopped, have the patient blow the nose to clear out all clots.
Assemble:
   - nasal speculum
   - cotton balls
   - suction/10F catheter tip
   - 4% topical lidocaine mixed with 1:1000 topical epinephrine or other combination anesthetic/vasoconstrictor.
   - bayonet forceps
   - cotton pledgets/dental roll
   - Vaseline gauze packing
   - lots of tissues or 4by4s

3. Put on the headlight and have the patient sit back. Place your hand on the patients forehead to prevent sudden jerks. Use the nasal speculum to spread the nares vertically and attempt to identify the bleeding source.

4. If bleeding is brisk, use the bayonet forceps to insert three cotton pledgets or dental rolls soaked in a mixture of lidocaine and epinephrine. The first goes on the floor of the nasal cavity, the second in the middle meatus, the third in the roof of the nasal cavity. Bleeding that does not stop after this maneuver may require posterior packing.

5. After 5 minutes, remove the packing and re-attempt to identify the site of the bleeding. Once the bleeding source is found, cauterize the area using silver nitrate sticks.

6. Have the patient sit around for a while after the bleeding has been stopped to ensure hemostasis has been obtained.

7. Bleeding that continues and is not posterior should be re-packed with soaked pledgets and left for another 5-10 minutes. If bleeding reoccurs after such time, pack the nose with vaseline gauze, put the patient on prophylactic antibiotics (Amoxicillin will do) and arrange for ENT follow up in 2 to 4 days.

8. Posterior bleeds or bleeds that continue despite anterior packing should get ENT consultation in the ED.

Eye

"Remember how little you know. Don't be afraid to say you don't know. Don't lay claim to superior knowledge." W.S. Thayer, MD 1928

Ocular complaints include foreign body, trauma, caustic injury, red/painful eye, lid problems and changes in visual acuity. The approach to each is the same with minor modifications:

Eye Examination

1. Except in cases of caustic or splash injury, test visual acuity before mucking around with the eye. Caustic injury or toxic exposures demand irrigation for at least 15 minutes before anything else.

2. Examine the orbit, pupils, extra-ocular motions, cornea, sclera. iris. Evert the upper lid with a Q-tip and retract both lids sufficiently to absolutely rule out any foreign body. Facilitate examination with anesthetic drops prn.

3. Slit-lamp examination.

4. Fluorescein stain for corneal abrasions.

5. Tonometry if increased intra-ocular pressure is suspected.

Red/Painful Eye

Conjunctivitis

Bacterial versus viral

Rx: gentamicin drops by day ointment by night.

Episcleritis.

Sub-conjunctival hemorrhage.

Acute angle closure glaucoma-increased intraocular pressure

Keratitis-inflammation or infection of the cornea.

Iritis/uveitis.

Foreign body (FB)

Anesthetize eye and remove FB.

Rule out corneal abrasion and penetrating injury.

Consider skull films to r/o intra-ocular fb.

Corneal abrasion

Apply gentamicin ointment.

Apply metal eye shield with compressive dressing.

Follow up with ophthalmology next day.

Corneal ulceration

Get ophthalmology involved right away.

Eye (continued)

Splash injury

May occur with alkali, acid or toxic compounds. The most serious of the three is alkali which can cause severe burns.

1. Initiate saline or LR irrigation for at least 15 minutes (or 2 liters) before examining the eye. Be sure to protect yourself from whatever material is involved.

2. Test tears with pH paper and continue irrigation until pH is 7-8.

3. Complete remainder of ocular exam and consult ophthalmology.

Lid Problems

Hordeolum (sty): painful swollen suppurative pustule on lid margin.
Chalazion: granulomatous and generally non-infected meibomian gland cyst.
Blepharitis: inflammation of the eyelid margin.
Dacryocystitis: infection of lacrimal sac.
Periorbital cellulitis: infection of eyelids.

Trauma

Blow out fracture with intraocular muscle entrapment.
Ruptured globe.
Lid laceration.
Posterior segment hemorrhage.
Retinal detachment.
Hyphema-blood in anterior chamber.

Acute Visual Loss or Acuity Change

Central retinal artery occlusion.
Central retinal vein occlusion.
Detached retina.
Vitreous hemorrhage.
Optic neuritis.
Giant cell arteritis.

NB: never prescribe or dispense anesthetic or steroid drops to patients going home. Always give ophthalmology a call when in doubt.

Foot and Ankle

Associated injuries include spinal, proximal fibular, and fifth metatarsal fractures.

1. History: document mechanism of injury. Delineate if inversion, eversion or axial forces were involved. Document past problems as sprains can become a chronic problem from lax ligaments. Is the patient able to bear weight? Inquire about pain in spine, proximal lower extremity and fifth metatarsal, which are frequent associated injuries. Td if laceration, abrasion, or open fracture.

2. Physical: check distal pulses and inspect condition of overlying skin. Begin at knee and work distally, palpating less tender areas first. Palpate spine, proximal fibula, and base of fifth metatarsal.

3. Radiology: (standard views)
    Ankle: AP, lateral and mortise views.
    Foot: AP, lateral and oblique.

Inversion injuries are most common and usually result in sprained lateral ligaments. Proximal 5th metatarsal fractures (Jones), avulsion fractures of the lateral malleolus and bimalleolar fractures may also occur.
Eversion injuries are also common, but because of the strength and elasticity of the medial (deltoid) ligament, sprains are less common. Fractures, dislocations and proximal fibula (Maisonneuve) fractures may also occur.
Axial loads may cause calcaneus and talus fractures as well as a host of other foot and ankle fractures.

Ankle Sprains: (negative X-ray) can be placed in either an ace wrap or sugar tong splint depending on severity. Rest, ice, compression and elevation aid healing. Weight bearing is begun once pain and swelling have subsided. Follow up with orthopedist in 7-10 days if not getting better.

Single malleolar fractures, complete ligament tears, Achilles tendon ruptures, distal tibia or fibular fractures, and foot fractures that represent stable, reduced joint injuries demand non-weight bearing, posterior or sugar-tong splinting, and follow-up in 2-3 days.

Bilateral/trimalleolar fractures, fracture dislocations, and open fractures require ED orthopedic consultation for consideration of early surgical intervention. Immobilize until definitive care can be arranged.

Non-displaced tarsal, metatarsal, and proximal phalanx fractures can be splinted, and made not-weight bearing, with early ortho follow-up. Displaced fractures should be seen by the orthopedist.

Distal phalangeal fractures get buddy-taped and placed in post-op shoe for cane walking and activity as tolerated. March (stress) fractures can be treated the same way.

Fractures

While definitive management of fractures is the purview of the orthopedist, the emergency physician minimizes complications, initiates therapy, and guides follow-up. For the novice, the most difficult part can be fracture nosology.

Definitions:

- Open vs. closed: is the skin over the fracture intact ?
- Transverse, oblique, spiral: direction of the fracture line ?
- Simple vs. Comminuted: two or multiple fragments.
- Displacement: position of the distal fragment with respect to the proximal one.
  - Valgus: away. Varus: towards the body.
  - Dorsal or posterior vs. volar or anterior.
  - Angulation: degree of deformity.
- Impaction: distal fragment driven into proximal one.
- Avulsion: bone pulled off where tendon or ligament inserts.
- Greenstick: disruption of one cortex with resultant angulation.
- Torus or Buckle: axial load causes cortex to wrinkle & form bump.
- Compound: old term for open fracture. Do not use.

Salter-Harris classification system: used to describe fractures involving epiphyseal (growth) plates.

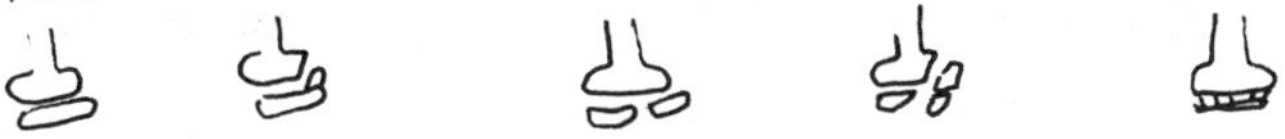

Type I (Best) | Type II | Type III | Type IV | Type V (Worst)

Eponyms:

- Barton: dorsal rim of the articular surface of the distal radius.
- Bennett: 2 fragment fracture of the articular surface of the proximal metacarpal.
- Boxer: fifth metacarpal.
- Colles: distal radius fracture with dorsal displacement.
- Galeazzi's: radial shaft fracture associated with distal radioulnar dislocation.
- Hangman's: pedicle(s) of C-2 from hyperextension.
- Hutchinson/Chauffeur: distal radial styloid.
- Jefferson: burst fracture of ring of C-1 from axial force.
- Jones: fracture of base of fifth metatarsal from inversion injury.
- Maissonneuve: proximal fibula fracture associated with ankle mortise disruption.
- Malgaigne: pelvic fracture with both anterior and posterior components.
- March: stress fracture of foot, generally proximal metatarsal.
- Monteggia: ulnar fracture associated with radial head dislocation.
- Neer: comminuted (3 or more fragment) fracture of proximal humerus.
- Rolando: >2 fragment interarticular fracture of the proximal, first metacarpal.
- Segond: vertical avulsion fracture of the lateral proximal tibia.
- Smith: a "reverse" Colles fracture.
- Tillaux: Salter III fracture of the anterolateral distal tibial epiphysis.

Fractures (continued)

General Management of Fractures: most serious complications of fractures result from the neurovascular damage incurred as a direct result of the injury, failure to immobilize adequately, or infection from an open fracture.

1. Examine and document distal pulses and examine color and temperature of extremity while saying hello.

2. Examine for open fracture by completely disrobing the affected extremity. If an open fracture exists remove any gross contamination, cover with sterile dressing and wet with saline.

3. Presence of open fracture or pulselessness demands immediate attention. Let your ER resident or attending know about the patient right away, *before* the x-ray. Urgent orthopedic consultation is also required. Document neurovascular exam before and after any manipulation.

4. In the absence of pulselessness or an open fracture, obtain the history while examining for deformity, changes in overlying skin, asymmetry, bony tenderness, range of motion in joints and sensation.

5. Examine patient for any associated injuries.

6. Tetanus immunization if indicated.

7. X-ray studies as warranted.

8. Document history, examination, x-ray findings, method of immobilization, analgesia prescribed and document and provide adequate follow up with primary care physician or orthopedist.

9. Patient instructions center around the RICE pneumonic:
    Rest-provide time off as appropriate.
    Ice-for 24-48 hours to minimize swelling.
    Compression-the splint should provide this.
    Elevation-keep injured part above the heart for 24-48hrs.

Frostbite

Like burns, the severity of injury is proportional to the duration of exposure and the temperature gradient between body and environment.

History: duration and type of exposure, comorbidity, history of prior frostbite, presence of Raynaud's disease. Psychiatric history and intoxication are common.

Physical: patients most often present with some degree of numbness, and affected areas appear white, yellow or mottled.

Management:

1. ABCs and initiate management of hypothermia. Establish IV access and urine output.

2. Avoid any possibility of refreezing after rewarming has begun, and avoid use of any mechanical means (i.e. rubbing) to rewarm parts.

3. Immerse in water between 40-43C. (104-109F).
Rewarming should continue until part feels right and erythema returns to distal extremity.

4. Provide adequate analgesia as pain will become severe.

5. Manipulate gently. Elevate extremity to avoid swelling and apply thin layer of topical aloe vera. Drain any blisters and apply sterile dressing.

6. Tetanus.

7. Consider NSAIDs and streptococcal prophylaxis.

GI Bleeding

Assure adequate airway and breathing (provide O_2 either 15L via FM or 6L via NC).

1. Assess circulation/degree of hypovolemia:
   BP, pulse, orthostatics, capillary refill, cool, clammy?
   Assess mental status.
   Cardiac monitor.
   Trendelenburg prn.
2. Volume resuscitation:
   Two to Six large bore IVs with NS or LR.
   Triple lumen catheters provide less volume than short 14G IVs.
3. Assess site of bleeding: Guaiac stool.
   Place NGT and lavage until clear.
4. Optimize milieu for thrombosis and package for admission:
   CBC, Chem7, PT/PTT, LFTs, Ca^{++}, Type&Cross 2-6units PRBCs.
   PCXR rule out impending CHF, intestinal perforation.
   H2 blocker.
   Correct coags with FFP and Vitamin K.
   Correct acidosis.
   Correct hypothermia.
   Consider DDAVP, vasopressin, Blakemore tube.
5. Rule out comorbidity:
   Rule out ischemia, and make sure that volume resuscitation is not throwing the patient into CHF.
6. History:
   Onset and duration. Melena vs. hematochezia.
   Coffee ground emesis.
   Past bleeds, ulcers, surgery, CA, aortic graft, liver disease.
   Use of ASA, NSAIDs, warfarin, anti-platelet agents
7. Consults:
   GI for possible emergent upper endoscopy.
   General Surgery to follow for possible emergent celiotomy.
   ICU.
8. Localize bleeding source: Angiogram, bleeding scan, endoscopy.
   Some Causes of GI Bleeding:

Upper:	Lower:
PUD	Diverticulosis
Gastritis	Angiodysplasia
Varices	CA/polyposis
Mallory-Weiss	Hemorrhoids/fissures
Esophagitis	UC/Crohn's

Hand

Disorders of the hand include fractures, dislocations, avulsions, lacerations, contusions, infections and tendon injuries, and constitute an entire surgical subspecialty. Referrals should be made early and often.

History: first remove all jewelry. Document mechanism or onset of problem, past problems with hand, dominance, past medical history and last tetanus.

Physical: exam hand held at rest, assess distal pulses and capillary refill, then inspect for breaks in skin, lacerations, contusions and deformity. Palpate for bony and soft tissue tenderness and test median, ulnar and radial nerves. Test tendons:

> Obvious injuries should not be stressed. Inability to extend each of the digits against resistance suggests extensor tendon injury. Inability to flex the finger at the DIP with the PIP held in extension suggests flexor digitorum profundus injury, while inability to flex at the PIP joint with the other fingers held in extension suggests flexor digitorum superficialis injury.

Radiology: AP, lateral and oblique views. Used to evaluate for fractures, tendon avulsions, soft tissue swelling and foreign bodies.

Some Disorders of the Hand

Lacerations: are best managed by experienced persons, but do well when prepped, copiously irrigated and meticulously repaired. Rule out foreign body or tendon injury and get plastics or ortho involved if in any doubt. Prophylactic antibiotics are recommended. Do not close bite wounds. See Wounds and Lacerations page 69.

Fractures: management is usually dictated by the amount of deformity present. Rotational deformity is tested by ensuring that all the flexed fingers line up and point to the base of the thumb. Any amount of rotational deformity, significant displacement or angulation, or articular involvement should prompt orthopedic consultation.

Infections: can lead to permanent disability. Admission for IV antibiotics is often necessary, although many can be managed as outpatients. Flexor tenosynovitis should be suspected in any patient with tenderness, pain on passive extension or fusiform swelling in a finger.

Felons: are infections of the pulp space of the hand, and form because fascial septa make internal drainage of the space difficult. They should be drained.

Paronychia: are infections of the skin surrounding the nail bed.

Subungual hematomas: occur from trauma and should be drained with a hot wire to relieve pain and pressure.

Headache

Treat pain and rule out serious pathology.

History: onset, provocation, quality, relief, severity, timing? Prior trauma, fever, sinus congestion, glaucoma? A history of migraines should be taken lightly if this episode is not characteristic of the patients past episodes. New or sudden onset HA, change in character, slowly evolving HA, or focal signs suggest serious pathology.

Vital signs.
Neuro: disks, visual fields, II-XII, sensory, motor, reflexes, cerebellar.
General: palpation of cranium, sinus tenderness, nuchal rigidity external ocular exam, photophobia. Tonometry.

Studies:
CT: without contrast to rule out intracerebral bleed, mass, or cerebral edema. No blood is seen in 15-25% of sub-arachnoid hemorrhage (SAH).
LP: r/o meningitis, encephalitis, SAH. Send first and last tubes for cell count to distinguish SAH from traumatic tap. Xanchromia is also useful if sxs >6 hours.
ESR: elevated in cases of cranial arteritis.
Sinus films.

<u>Serious</u>
Sub arachnoid hemorrhage
Meningitis/encephalitis
Cranial arteritis
Traumatic/Non-traumatic bleeds
- Epidural hematoma
- Subdural hematoma
- Intraparenchymal bleed

Glaucoma
Mass/tumor
Toxic/Metabolic
Hypercarbia, hypoxia
Malignant HTN

<u>Not so serious</u>
Migraines
- Classic
- Common
- Ophthalmic

Cluster headache
Trigeminal neuralgia
Sinusitis
Tension headache
Post LP headache
Caffeine responsive
TMJ syndrome

Treatment of Migraine: IV is better than IM. Prochlorperazine controls nausea and vomiting, and is used to prevent the nausea associated with DHE or narcotics.
- Prochlorperazine 10mg slow IV over 2 minutes and,
- DHE 0.75-1.0 mg slow IV or IM or,
- Meperidine 50-100mg slow IV or IM or,
- Ketorolac 60mg IM (avoid in any potential bleed).

Treatment of headaches other than migraine is similar, although DHE may not be as effective. Failure to respond to therapy is worrisome and further studies should be considered. Be cautious about diagnosing drug seeking behavior.
Follow up with primary physician or neurologist is mandatory.

Heat Related Illness

Patients are most commonly brought to the ED on the hottest days, although milder temperatures can cause heat related illness in poorly acclimatized individuals or in extremes of humidity. Symptoms range from mild heat cramps with normal body temperature to coma in full blown heat stroke.

Because evaporation is the most effective cooling process, cooling is undertaken with spray bottle and fans. Shivering produces heat and should be avoided during the cooling process.

Clinical Syndromes

Heat Cramps: are characterized by painful muscle spasm and are common during athletic events. They are thought to occur from hyponatremia in individuals who replace free water, but not salt losses. Body temperature may be normal or elevated. Rest and use of PO or IV isotonic fluids is the mainstay of treatment. Instruct patients to replace lost fluids with balanced electrolyte solutions.

Heat Exhaustion: is characterized by headache, weakness, dizziness, nausea, vomiting, or syncope, but sensorium is otherwise clear. Treatment consist of cooling the patient, IV or PO fluids and rest and observation.

Heat Stroke: is characterized by mental status changes in association with elevated body temperature (>41°C). Shock, airway compromise, seizures, DIC, rhabdomyolysis, arrhythmias, and renal failure may occur. Rapid cooling and supportive care including ABCs is necessary.

1. ABCs: airway as appropriate, obtain IV access and initiate cool IVF bolus of 1-2 liters.

2. Institute rapid cooling by disrobing the patient and spraying with cool, not cold water and positioning fans onto the patient.

3. Check electrolytes, glucose, CPK, Mg^{++}, Ca^{++} and CBC.

Hip, Leg and Knee

"I've fallen and I can't get up!"

Injuries to the lower extremity are common, especially in the elderly and the athletic. The most important factor to determine is whether the patient is able to walk; non-ambulatory patients generally cannot go home.

Consider giving something for pain while initiating studies.

Hip injuries: most commonly occur during athletic activity. In the elderly they occur in falls. The classic presentation of hip fracture is an elderly woman who has "fallen and can't get up," who presents with a foreshortened and externally rotated leg. Consider head, neck and other injuries. Establish IV, check the pedal pulses, and send to radiology. It is best to avoid manipulating the joint until fracture is ruled out.

Radiology: (standard views)
- AP: often of the pelvis to compare with the other side.
- Lateral: taken with patient supine.
  - Inspect Shenton's line and trabecular network for subtle fractures.

Slipped capital femoral epiphyses, Legg-Perthes disease and toxic synovitis are causes of hip pain in kids. In absence of positive findings, consider orthopedic consultation and referral.

Femur fractures: demand immediate attention and immobilization in a traction splint. Get ortho involved right away. Establish IV access and get x-rays. Associated injuries are common. Patients can loose a significant amount of blood into the thigh.

Knee injuries: arise from both valgus and varus stresses applied to the knee. Ligamentous injuries are more common than fractures. Chondral damage can occur, especially from twisting injuries. Test both collateral ligaments by holding the knee in slight flexion and moving leg in either direction. Test the anterior cruciate ligament using the anterior drawer test.

Radiology: (standard views)
- AP, Obliques
- Cross-table lateral: may show fat-fluid level if hemarthrosis is present.
- Patella: include axial (sunrise) view.

Most knee injuries are ligamentous and can be placed in a knee immobilizer with crutches or weight bearing as tolerated and referred for orthopedic follow up. Rest, ice, compression, and elevation will reduce swelling and pain. Fractures about the knee should prompt orthopedic consultation in the ED or long leg splinting, non-weight bearing and early follow up.

Knee dislocation is an emergency, get help.

Patella dislocation is much less urgent and is usually reduced by the time you see the patient.

Hypercalcemia

Etiology:

45%	Malignancy: breast, lung, prostate, multiple myeloma.
45%	Primary hyperparathyroidism.
10%	Drugs: thiazide, lithium, and estrogens, milk+alkali.
Others	TB, sarcoid, hypoadrenalism, immobilization, genetic.

Reference range: 8.5-10.5 mg/dl. [>12 panic]

Corrected Calcium(mg/dl) = Measured Calcium + 0.8 [4 - albumin]

Symptoms and Signs:

CNS: weakness, lethargy, confusion, decreased reflexes, coma.
GI: nausea, vomiting, constipation, PUD, pancreatitis.
CV: HTN, QT shortening.
Renal: polyuria, nephrolithiasis, nephrocalcinosis.

Treatment: should be based on the extent of symptoms.

1. Saline is the first line of therapy. In patients without history of CHF, 2-4 liters of saline maybe given a day to promote caluresis. Begin in the ED with a hefty bolus to restore intravascular volume. Be gentle in patients with possible CHF.

2. Furosemide is used to promote further caluresis in patients with very high calcium levels. Volume should be restored with saline initially, and potassium and other electrolytes need to be checked and monitored frequently.

3. Calcitonin (salmon or human) generally causes the calcium to drop an additional one-half point in a few hours, and is the only other drug that should be considered in the ED. 4U/kg IV/IM/SQ. An initial 1U skin test is given initially.

Hyperkalemia

Therapy is dictated by degree of K^+ elevation and EKG changes.

Reference range:	3.3-5.0 meq/L	normal
	5.0-6.0 meq/L	mild
	6.0-7.0 meq/L	moderate
	>7.0, symptoms, EKG changes	severe

Symptoms: numbness, weakness, decreased reflexes, cardiac arrest.

EKG: tall, thin, "peaked" T waves, QT interval shortening, PR interval prolongation, ST segment depression, QRS widening, P wave disappearance, sine-wave pattern, v-fib, asystole.

Treatment: initiate continuous cardiac monitoring.

1. Antagonize membrane effects of potassium.
   Calcium Gluconate (10%) 10ml over 5 minutes. (In cases of Digoxin use, administer over 30 minutes).
2. Shift potassium into cells.
   Sodium Bicarbonate (7.5%) 1 Amp IV over 5 min. (Helpful when acidosis is causing K^+ shifts).
   Glucose (D50%) One Amp over 5 minutes plus Insulin (regular) 5-10 Units IVP. Consider 10 units IV in diabetics. Follow glucose levels.
3. Reduce total body potassium pool.
   Exchange resin (Kayexalate) 30gm PO in 100cc 20% sorbitol.
   In patients not taking PO, 50gm PR in 200cc 20% sorbitol is be administered by enema.
   Furosemide 40mg IVP with K^+ free IVF.
   Dialysis: in cases of extremely high K^+ levels despite use of exchange resins or in patients with impaired renal function.
   Monitor other electrolytes, especially Mg^{++}, Ca^{++}.
4. Consider etiologies.

Volume depletion/dehydration	Hypoaldosteronism
Renal failure	RTA Type 4
Acidosis	Tissue catabolism
Exogenous K^+ administration	Digoxin toxicity
Pseudohyperkalemia (hemolysis)	Beta-blockers
K^+ sparing diuretics:	Succinylcholine
ACE inhibitor, spironolactone	

Hypothermia

Aphorism: *"They're not dead until they're warm and dead."*

Mild:	< 36°C (97°F).
Moderate:	< 34°C (93°F).
Severe:	< 30°C (86°F).

Precipitating factors: drugs, EtOH, trauma, homelessness, psychiatric disease.

Management:

1. Avoid rough handling of the patient as this may precipitate VF.

2. Remove wet or damp garments, apply warm packs to neck, groin, and armpits.

3. Administer warm humidified O2.

4. Apply cardiac monitor for arrhythmias.

5. Establish an IV and begin warm IVF.

6. Check core temperature. Not all thermometers register cold temperatures.

7. Mild cases may be managed with blankets and passive rewarming alone. Moderate cases require active external rewarming. Severe cases demand internal rewarming with warm peritoneal lavage, pleural lavage, and gastric lavage in addition to all external measures.

Joint Pain

ED evaluation centers around tapping any joint suspected of infection.
Only septic arthritis can do the patient much harm.

1. Consider whether the patient has a monarticular, polyarticular, non-articular or traumatic cause for joint pain:

Monarticular	Polyarticular	Non-articular	Traumatic
Septic Osteoarthritis Gout Pseudogout	Gonococcal Rheumatoid Lyme	Bursitis Tendinitis Cellulitis* Hemarthrosis	Fracture Sprain Dislocation

2. If septic, gonococcal, or hemarthritic causes cannot be ruled out by the establishment of another diagnosis, then the joint must be tapped. Consider tapping every joint that comes in with acute non-traumatic pain, even in the absence of redness, swelling or fever.

3. Consider radiographs to evaluate for articular destruction, soft tissue swelling, foreign body or gas.

4. Perform arthrocentesis under sterile prep, drapes, local infiltration with lidocaine with a #18 gauge needle in large joints and a #20 in smaller joints.

5. Remove as much fluid as possible. Dab a small amount on a glass slide, a small amount on a culture swab and divide the remaining portion between purple and red pediatric blood tubes. If fluid is especially sparse priority should be:

Gram Stain > Culture > Crystals > Cell Count > Glucose.

6. Joint Fluid Analysis

	Normal	Noninflammatory	Inflammatory	Septic
Gram Stain	-	-	-	+
Culture	-	-	-	+
Crystals	-	-	+/-	-
Cell Count	>200	200-2000	2000-50,000	>50,000
% Polys	>25%	>25%	>50%	>75%
Glucose	=serum	=serum	>25mg/dl	<25mg/dl

7. Treatment/Disposition
Septic arthritis: admission for IV antibiotics: nafcillin, first generation cephalosporin or ampicillin/sulbactam if gram+ organism, for gram(-) organism or if GC suspected, then ceftriaxone.
Gout/Inflammatory: NSAID at maximum dose for a few days then reduce to a maintenance dose. Consider colchicine. Follow up with internist.
Non-inflammatory: Acetaminophen 1000 PO Q4-6 PRN.

Kidney Stones

Renal colic is relatively easy to diagnose in a person with a history of stones who comes to the ER writhing from flank pain that radiates to the groin with urine that dips positive for blood. You may be asked: "how much do you want to give him," even before you see the patient. A quick history and physical to rule out a surgical abdomen (peritoneal signs) should allay some anxiety about giving narcotics to a patient with abdominal pain.

Get a UA and consider nephrolithiasis in every patient with abdominal pain.

1. History: previous history of stones, renal disease, or causes for hypercalcuria or hyperuricuria. Onset, severity and quality, character, and nature of pain. Symptoms of peritoneal inflammation should lead away from the diagnosis of renal colic.

2. Physical: abdominal exam variable, but any patient with rebound or severe guarding should be worked up as a surgical abdomen and not renal colic even if prior history of stones and hematuria are present. Pelvic to r/o adnexal tenderness from ovarian cyst, or torsion. Appendicitis? Think about AAA and rule it out.

3. Analgesia: as soon as the diagnosis of renal colic is settled.
    - Meperidine 50-100mg IV with Promethazine 12.5mg IV.
    - Begin IVF with NS or LR at 150-200cc/hr unless h/o CHF.

4. Labs: CBC with differential, UA, C+S. SMA7 if vomiting severe or if IVP planned.

5. KUB: indicated in most patients with suspected kidney stones; rule out pregnancy first.

6. IVP: confirms the diagnosis and rules out complete obstruction. May be avoided in patients with resolution of symptoms and strong suspicion of diagnosis.

7. Disposition:
    - Home:
        - Urologic follow-up within one or two days.
        - Provide adequate analgesics, anti-emetics.
        - Strain urine and save particulate matter for the urologist.
    - Admission:
        - Fever, WBC>15,000, infected urine.
        - Intractable pain or vomiting.
        - Significant hematuria.
        - Ureteral perforation.
        - Extremes of age.
        - High grade obstruction.
        - Pre-existing renal disease or solitary kidney.

Motor Vehicle Accident

Patients come in on a back-board, hopefully with adequate cervical spine immobilization (hard collar). Don't let the paramedics leave before talking with them. Major trauma victims are quickly recognized in the field, your job is to rule out occult injury in less traumatized patients.

1. Airway with C-spine Immobilization:
   Inspect oropharynx for blood, avulsed teeth other injuries.
   Check that C-collar fits and patient is secured to board.
2. Breathing:
   Assess depth, rate and symmetry. Auscultate bilaterally.
   Palpate thorax for sternal and rib contusions.
3. Circulation:
   Assess VSSs and control any hemorrhage.
4. Deficit:
   Patient should cooperate and communicate pain and injury.
   Assess motor strength and sensory exam in U/L extremities.
5. Exposure:
   Abdominal exam-tenderness, hematoma, consider splenic injury.
   Pelvis assessed by pressing down and in on hips. Look for other injuries.
   Cover open wounds with saline soaked sterile gauze or other dressing.
   Immobilize any possible fractures.

Any patient who fails the ABCDEs, has unstable vitals, or has changing mental status should be coded up to a trauma. Get help immediately.

6. History:

__yo M/F (un)belted driver/(front/back seat)passenger of a (air-bag equipped) make of car traveling at __mph hitting a (or hit from (location)) +/- loss of consciousness for (time). Windshield, steering wheel damage, condition of car. Condition of other occupants. PMH, medications, allergies. Any possibility of pregnancy??? If mechanism is significant, broken windshield or steering wheel, or other occupants dead, make sure some experienced eyes look at your patient with you early on.

7. C-spine series: any patient with neck pain, neurologic symptoms, spinous tenderness, or significant mechanism.

8. Further studies:
   HCT: LOC at scene, any change in MS since accident, mechanism.
   CXR: adequate for ribs in most cases but T-spine is necessary for evaluation of thoracic back pain.
   Aortogram: if widened medistinum or significant mechanism.
   Spine films: if significant pain or tenderness.
   AP Pelvis: if tender, painful or altered sensorium.
   Extremities: as indicated.
9. Once studies are complete, deal with fractures, lacerations and abrasions. Td.

Myocardial Infarction

Every possible therapy should be instituted, or at least considered, prior to transfer to the CCU. Therapy is very institution-depedent. Learn the local dogmas before meeting your first acute MI patient.

1. Before saying hello:
   O_2 at 4L via NC, IV access, Cardiac monitor, Pulse oximeter, Vitals, EKG.

2. History: call for old EKGs. Be brief.
   Prior MI, h/o CHF, prior cardiac therapy and interventions.
   Pain: onset duration, quality, radiation, intensity.
   Associated symptoms: SOB, diaphoresis, lightheadedness.
   Cardiac risk factors: DM, HTN, Tobacco, FH, Cholesterol.
   Medications. Eligibility and contraindications to thrombolytics.

3. Physical: VSSs, JVD, Carotid bruits, $S_1S_2S_3S_4$, murmurs, rales.
   Rectal prior to heparin or thrombolytics.

4. Therapy:
   ASA 325mg *chewed* in the ED.

   NTG 0.4mg sublingual q5minutes times three. After three sublingual nitroglycerine tablets, if still having pain and not hypotensive, begin:
   NTG (100mg/500cc D5W) at 5-10ug/min and titrate to pain-free, keeping SBP>90-110.

   Heparin 5000U bolus then (20,000U in 500cc D5W) @ 1000U/hr.

   MSO_4 1-2mg IV q5min until calm for pain and anxiety.

   Thrombolytic. If contraindicated, arrange for PTCA.

   Consider early **beta-blocker** if tachycardiac and/or BP stable, once NTG titrated, MSO_4 and lidocaine have been decided upon.

   Consider **Magnesium** 1-2 gm IV bolus then 0.5-1 gm/hr.
   Routine prophylactic use of Lidocaine is no longer recommended.

5. Studies: CBC, SMA7, Cardiac Enzymes, PT/PTT, Mg^{++}, UA, PCXR.

Avoid IM injections, foley, and ABGs in patients who may get thrombolytics.

Overdose

Antidotes do not replace adequate supportive care of the patient.

ED management occurs in four phases: stabilization, history, gastric decontamination then administration of antidotes. If the patient is awake and can talk he has passed the ABCs, (although he may not be able to in ten minutes). After the first three steps, consult the poison center. Always send acetaminophen level with tox screen.

Stabilization:

1. Airway with cervical spine stabilization.
2. Breathing: O_2, rate, depth, and character of resp.
3. Circulation: blood pressure and pulse rate.
4. IV Access: Draw tubes for labs and begin IVF.
   NS or LR if BP low, pulse high, or
   D5W KVO if BP normal or high.
5. Naloxone 2mg IVP.
6. D50 one amp (100ml).
7. Thiamine 100mg IVP.
8. Consider Flumazenil for benzodiazepine OD.
9. Call for EKG, C-spine (if neck injury suspected).
10. Rectal temperature.

History & Physical: look for clues to what was ingested. Rule out trauma. Substances, exact time? Psychiatric history, previous attempts, meds? Think about where the ingestion took place. If the patient was at home, think about what may have been co-ingested. Suicidal patients have no motivation to tell the truth.
Pupils, mucous membranes, lacrimation , salivation, sweating, dry axillae, bowel sounds, urine in bladder? Toxicologic syndromes are hard to remember, think about parasympathetic vs. sympathetic signs.

Gastric Decontamination: If patient is awake and will stay that way, then insert hose, lavage, and put charcoal down before pulling hose out. If the patient is groggy, protect the airway before putting the hose down.

11. Place patient in left lateral decubitus position.
12. Lavage using 36-40F orogastric hose (16-28F in children).
13. Activated Charcoal (AC)
    1-2 gm/kg dissolved in 250cc/30gm juice or water.

Remember that naloxone and flumazenil may have shorter half-lives than the drugs they are antagonizing.

Psych

"A man said to the universe: "Sir, I exist!"
"However," replied the universe, "the fact has not created in me a sense of obligation."
Stephen Crane, 1899.

Interns frequently hit the phone as soon as the patient hits the door. If a patient walked in asking to talk to a surgeon, would you call the surgeon before speaking to the patient? Get the history. While talking with the patient consider if the patient will need to be committed or if he or she simply needs to be offered the chance to come in. Do not exchange pathologies with the patient. Rule out organic causes of delirium: pulse-ox, lytes, etc.

History: What brought the patient in the ED?
- Substance use and abuse: quantify amount and recent change in habit.
- Past history of psychiatric hospitalizations: list if few.
- Suicidality/Homicidality: thought, plan, attempts.
- Psychiatric meds: antipsychotic, Li^+, antidepressants, sedatives.
- Medical conditions and non-psychiatric medications.

Mental Status Exam:
Level of consciousness, general appearance, demeanor, affect. Level of vigilance and attention span. Presence or absence of hallucinations, delusions or other persecutory thoughts. Memory to recent and distant events. Cognitive ability: calculations, proverbs. Reasoning, judgment, insight.

Physical Exam: Quick survey of heart, lungs, abdomen and back. Look for signs of exposure or abuse.

Labs: depends on institution. CBC, SMA7, SMA12, Tox screen, RPR, EtOH, Thyroid Profile.

Agitated patients:
1. First and foremost protect yourself. Don't go in by yourself, and stay by the door. Avoid arguments and don't try to reason; just leave.
2. Call security and get as many people involved as you can. Many patients back down when faced with a mob.
3. Restrain patient only if a threat to self or others.
4. Lorazepam: 2mgIV Q5min or 5mg IM Q20min -or-
   Haloperidol 5mg IM Q10 until calm. Watch the VSS.

Seizures

Seizures in adults are idiopathic or associated with EtOH withdrawal, trauma, metabolic disorders, CVAs or tumors. Unless a patient has a clear history of primary seizure disorder or EtOH abuse, work-up is mandatory.

Seizures in kids are either febrile, idiopathic, chronic, or associated with CNS infections, metabolic derangements, or toxins. History and physical is often enough to delineate their cause.

1. Provide an adequate airway with a nasal trumpet and administer O_2.

2. Assess breathing and augment as necessary. Ventilation is especially poor during the clonic phase.

3. Attach pulse-ox, cardiac monitor, and establish IV access.

4. If the seizure began in the ED, it will probably stop on its own.

5. Benzodiazepines are used to terminate prolonged seizures.
    Lorazepam 2-4mg (0.05-0.15mg/kg in children)
        Q2-5min IV prn.
    Diazepam 5mg (0.2-0.3 mg/kg in children) Q5min IV prn.
        (Up to 5-6 doses may be tried, continue to manage
        the ABCs).

6. Load with Phenytoin (Dilantin) 15-20mg/kg IV at a rate no greater than 1mg/kg/min or 50mg/min whichever is less. Loading dilantin orally guarantees the patient will seize again.

7. Phenobarbital 20mg/kg IV at a rate no faster than 50mg/min may be added if seizures continue despite Phenytoin. Watch for hypotension and respiratory depression.

8. Paraldehyde and general anesthesia are treatments of last resort.

Shock/Hypotension

Shock is defined as inadequate cellular perfusion. Hypotension is low BP. Treatment of either must be initiated rapidly and be directed to the underlying cause. While etiologies for shock are defined according to mechanism i.e. hypovolemic, cardiogenic and distributive shock, a stepped care approach is used when the diagnosis is uncertain.

1. Before anything else, consider airway, breathing and administer O2.

2. Establish IV access and attach cardiac monitor, pulse-ox and BP cuff. Place patient in Trendellenberg position. Initiate IVF bolus.

3. Order EKG and PCXR and perform a quick heart and lung exam looking for murmurs, crackles, pneumothorax, and JVD.

Now consider The Elements of Circulation: RRPAC:

Rate: a ventricular rate between 60-100 is best, although rates between 100 and 150 generally cause CHF and not hypotension. Atropine 0.5 - 1.0 mg IV for bradycardia. Also for symptomatic bradycardia, apply external pacer at 100bpm and turn up amps until it captures. If tachycardia is the problem, consider cardioversion or slowing the ventricular response (watch out: if unstable, use electricity, not negative inotropes).

Rhythm: if the ventricular rate is between 60-130, A-V dissociation is unlikely to be the problem. However, some patients need their atrial kick to provide adequate cardiac output. In the acute situation, make sure that the ventricular response is appropriate.

Preload: fill the pump before whipping it. The most common mistake is to administer pressors to a patient before adequate volume resuscitation. In all cases a fluid challenge should be the next line of therapy unless the patient is known to be volume overloaded. Begin with crystaloid (NS or LR) and use colloid or blood as necessary. Consider anaphylaxis.

Afterload: once the pump is full, (wedge pressure 12-16) initiate pressors. Remember that increasing afterload increases cardiac work. Dopamine is the first line agent because it increases both afterload and contractility and is easily titrated. Begin at 5ug/kg/min and titrate to keep SBP > 90. Epinephrine, norepinephrine and phenylephrine increase afterload as well.

Contractility: dobutamine and amrinone further increase contractility, but also decrease afterload, and thus are not first line agents in hypotension. Correct acidosis.

Etiologies:
Cardiogenic: MI, arrhythmia, drug depression, valve abnormality, cardiomyopathy, hypothermia.
Hypovolemic: hemorrhage, dehydration, burns, intestinal obstruction, pancreatitis.
Distributive: sepsis, anaphylaxis, hypo-oncotic, spinal cord transection.
Obstructive: PE, tamponade, tension pneumothorax, aortic stenosis.

Shoulder

The shoulder is the most freely mobile joint in the body. Stability is sacrificed for range of motion. Shoulder injuries include AC separations, clavicular fractures, shoulder dislocations and proximal humerus fractures.

1. History: mechanism of injury, anterior, posterior, or longitudinal forces; past or chronic subluxations, dislocations.

2. Physical: distal pulses; motor and sensory evaluation; obvious deformity. Palpate sternoclavicular joint and clavicle along its length, note presence or absence of step-off/ tenderness at AC joint, note position that patient holds shoulder, test ROM of shoulder to point of pain, and palpate scapula.

3. Radiology: (standard views)
   AP view in neutral position plus,
   AP with internal rotation plus,
   Lateral trans-thoracic (aka. scapular Y) view -or-,
   Axillary view.

AC Separation: can occur from a fall or direct blow to shoulder.
Grade I (sprain): incomplete tear of ligaments.
Tender AC joint with normal X-ray.
Grade II (subluxation): disrupted AC ligament but coracoclavicular (CC) ligament intact. X-rays may be negative or show AC separation less than 50% of the width of clavicle.
Grade III: complete AC and CC ligament disruption. X-rays show AC joint separation with clavicle displaced upward >50% of its diameter.

For grade I and II separations: apply sling for 10 days to 3 weeks, RICE, analgesia, early ROM exercises and ortho follow up with return to activity as tolerated. Grade III injuries should receive 6 weeks of immobilization and early ortho follow up for possible operative repair.

Clavicular Fracture: is the most common fracture in kids. They usually heal well, but severely displaced fractures should prompt orthopedic consultation to rule out vessel injury or fragment erosion through the skin. Treatment consists of immobilization with a sling and swathe or figure of eight bandage, RICE, analgesics, and ortho follow up.

Shoulder Dislocations: >90% are anterior. A scapular Y or axial view is required to confirm the diagnosis. Check neurovascular status and film all patients prior to manipulation. For anterior dislocations, IV analgesia is used for ED reduction. Check NV status, obtain films post reduction, and sling for 2-4 weeks with RICE. analgesics, and orthopedic follow-up. Posterior dislocations get ED orthopedic consultation.

Humeral Fractures: get ED orthopedic consultation.

Sickle Cell Crisis

Patients may be HbSS, HbSBeta-thalassemia, or HbSC. Quite rarely, sickle cell trait (HbAS) patients may present in painful crisis.

Management is aimed at ruling out infection or aplastic crisis, while providing volume repletion and relieving pain.

Contact the patient's hematologist for additional guidance.

1. Oxygen 2-4 lpm

2. IVF NS or 1/2NS at 150 to 200 cc/hr. Monitor for fluid overload.

3. History: onset of crisis, typical or atypical, location of pain. Precipitating factors, recent ED visits. Symptoms of infection: fever, cough, ST, otitis media, urinary symptoms. Consider PID.

4. Physical: brief, looking for signs of infection.

5. Narcotics: Patients often have a good idea how much narcotic will be necessary- this does not imply drug seeking behavior. IV narcotics offer slightly quicker relief, but patients experience a "rush," which many feel is inappropriate in patients requiring heavy narcotic use. Avoid Meperidine, which has a metabolite that can cause seizures, in favor of Morphine IV or SQ. Promethazine may be added for nausea 12.5mg IV or 25mg IM.

6. Laboratory/Studies: CBC, reticulocyte count-to evaluate for possible infection, severe anemia, and to rule out aplastic crisis.
   UA to r/o UTI. CXR to rule out infiltrate.
   Reticulocyte Index = Reticulocyte count * [patients Hct / normal Hct]

7. Patients should be offered a fixed number of injections at 2-3 hour intervals at the end of which time they will need to decide if they can go home with a small supply of pain meds, or if they need to be admitted for additional pain control. Multiple ED visits mandate consideration of early admission.

STDs/Genital Tract Infections

"No matter how exemplary one's conduct may be, there is always a chance, which is not so remote as many people imagine, for an accidental infection. Many women are infected by their husbands, who had the disease and thought they were cured before they were married." Benjamin E. Washburn, MD 1930.

Get a pregnancy test. Avoid doxycycline, ciprofloxacin, tetracycline, and metronidazole in pregnancy, and avoid TMP/SMX in the third trimester.

Syphilis: Treponema pallidum.
Dx: 1°: painless "chancre" 1wk-3mo post exposure.
2°: maculopapular rash on palms and soles.
3°: latent, disseminated, neuro, gummas.
Rx: 1°,2°,3°<1yr-PEN G (benzathine) 2.4 MU IM once.
3°>1yr-PEN G (benzathine) 2.4 MU IM Qwk times 3.
Neuro-PEN G (aq) 2-4MU IM qd for 10-14 days.

Gonorrhea: Neisseria gonorrhea.
Dx: Drip, discharge, friable cervix, sore throat, PID.
May be asymptomatic.
Rx: Cervicitis,urethritis,pharyngitis,proctitis:
Ceftriaxone 250mg IM once + rx for chlamydia.
Ophthalmia: Ceftriaxone 1gm IM daily for 5days.

Non-gonococcal urethritis/cervicitis: Chlamydia/Ureaplasma.
Dx: Drip, discharge (little), cervicitis.
Rx: Doxycycline 100mg PO BID for 7 days -or-
Tetracycline 500mg PO QID for 7 days -or-
Erythromycin 500mg PO QID for 7 days.

Lymphogranuloma venereum (LGV): C. Trachomatis.
Dx: Painless ulcer, tender, swollen, fluctuant, adherent inguinal nodes, draining nodes, fever, HA, joint pain.
Rx: Doxycycline 100mg PO BID for 21 days -or-
Tetracycline 500mg PO QID for 21 days -or-
Erythromycin 500mg PO QID for 21 days.

Chancroid: Hemophilus ducreyi.
Dx: Shallow, painful, non-indurated ulcer, with reddish border. Tender, swollen, matted inguinal nodes (bubo) with possible draining sinuses.
Rx: Ceftriaxone 250mg IM once -or-
Erythromycin 500mg PO QID for 7 days -or-
Ciprofloxacin 500mg PO BID for 3 days.

Granuloma Inguinale: Calymmatobacterium granulomatis (Donovan b).
Dx: Painless nodule that evolves into a granulomatous mass.
Lymphadenopathy noticeably absent.
Rx: Doxycycline 100mg PO BID or Tetracycline 500mg PO QID until healed -or- TMP/SMX BID until healed.

STDs/Genital Tract Infections (continued)

Trichomonas: Trichomonas vaginalis.

Dx: Urethritis, vaginitis: copious yellow/green, frothy malodorous discharge. Wet prep (+) for trichomonad.

Rx: Metronidazole 2GM PO once or 500mg PO BID for 7 days.

Bacterial Vaginosis: Gardnerella vaginalis, bacteroides, others.

Dx: Copious, white to yellow, discharge with fishy (amine) odor on KOH prep. Wet prep (+) for clue cells.

Rx: Metronidazole 500mg PO BID for 7 days.

Candidiasis: Candidial organisms.

Dx: Cottage cheese like, white to yellow discharge. KOH prep shows non septate hyphae.

Rx: Clotrimazole 100mg vaginal suppository QHS for 7 days or 2 100mg supp QHS for 3 days or Clotrimazole 1% cream: 1 applicator full (5gm)QHS for 7-14 days.

Herpes: Herpes simplex virus Types II and I.

Dx: Multiple, painful, small, ulcerated erythematous or crusted lesions. (+)Tzank prep of ulcer material.

Rx: Acyclovir 200mg PO 5x/day for 10days if no history of prior infection, 5 days if secondary infection.

Genital Warts: human papilloma virus.

Dx: Small, raised, warts on cervix or penis which turn white on application of acetic acid.

Rx: Referral to OB/GYN or Urologist for definitive rx.

Epididimitis/orchitis: GC, Chlamydia, Enterobacteriaceae, mumps.

Dx: Painful, tender, scrotum with fever, r/o testicular torsion and consider mumps orchitis/epididimitis. Culture urethral discharge or urine.

Rx: Based of suspicion of GC/Chlamydia would rx for above or for coliforms with TMP/SMX double strength BID or Ciprofloxacin 500mg PO BID for 14 days.

Prostatitis: enterobacteriaceae, other colonic organisms.

Dx: Fever, chills, dysuria, frequency, tender prostate. Urine cx usually (+).

Rx: TMP/SMX double strength BID or Norfloxacin 400mg PO BID or Ciprofloxacin 500 PO BID for 14 days.

Endometritis: postpartum-bacteroides, group B strep, colonic organisms. Late postpartum-chlamydia. Post abortion-r/o retained prod. of conception.

Dx: Fever, chills, abdominal pain postpartum.

Rx: Admit to OB/GYN for IV antibiotics.

Stridor

Stridor is caused by obstruction of large airways and can herald sudden airway closure.

1. Provide cool humidified O_2 without inducing additional anxiety. Parents may hold the child and the O_2 set-up.
2. Pulse-ox may be helpful, but avoid any invasive procedures.
3. Observe for tachypnea, cyanosis, unresponsiveness or hypoxemia. Do not test gag. Get help and assemble airway instruments for transfer to OR for intubation.
4. In stable patients, a soft tissue lateral neck may be helpful.

Epiglottitis: rule out in all cases of stridor. Symptoms arise rapidly and include fever, toxic appearance, drooling, dysphagia, and extended posture. Children between 2-7 years are most commonly affected, and infection is caused by H. flu. Diagnosis is confirmed by noting swollen epiglottis or "thumb" sign on lateral soft tissue neck film. Definitive management consists of endotracheal intubation under OR conditions, ICU admission, and parenteral antibiotics.

Croup: is an inflammatory disorder of the larynx associated with viral URI. It is most common in children between 6mo-3yrs, in the fall and winter, and in the early morning hours. High fevers, dysphagia, drooling and systemic toxicity are rare. Patients benefit from humidified O_2 and Racemic Epinephrine (2.25%) 0.05cc/kg (0.25cc to 0.5cc) in 2.5ccNS via nebulizer. Parenteral steroids are used for severe cases. Rebound may occur with racemic epinephrine so patients must be admitted.

Croup Score 0-10

Observation	0	1	2
Insp. Breath Sounds	Normal	Rhonchi	Delayed
Stridor	None	I	I/E
Cough	None	Hoarse	Bark
Retractions	None	Suprasternal	Intercostal
Cyanosis	None	Room Air	On40% O_2

Bacterial Tracheitis: is often indistinguishable from epiglottitis on clinical grounds. S.aureus is causative. Patients present with stridor, fever, toxic appearance and increased WBC count. The diagnosis is frequently suspected when a patient with normal lateral soft tissue films fails to improve with standard croup therapy.

Foreign Body: in the airway or the esophagus, when large enough, can cause airway obstruction. For radiolucent objects, fluoroscopy may be helpful. Consider in any patient, previously well, who presents with sudden onset of stridor.

Other Causes: include peritonsillar abscess, retro-pharyngeal abscess, traumatic, congenital and neoplastic disorders.

Syncope

Patients with syncope and near-syncope can present at any age. Since the work-up of syncope consists of many tests to rule out life threatening etiologies, patients are frequently admitted.

1. Initial Management:
   ABCs.
   Neurologic deficit.
   EKG to rule out MI/Arrhythmia.
   Guaiac/NGT? to rule out GIB.
   Pregnancy test in every female of child bearing age.

2. History: helpful in differentiating between seizure and syncope: onset, aura, duration of unconsciousness, tonic-clonic activity, loss of bowel/bladder, witnesses. Pay particular attention to medications, especially changes in dose or frequency as well as history of cardiac or peripheral vascular disease.

3. Physical: BP (both arms) and orthostatics, cardiac auscultation, carotid bruits, signs of PVD, guaiac. Auscultation with valsalva for IHSS in young weight-lifters.

4. Studies: include EKG, cardiac monitoring, CBC, glucose pulse-ox, echo, Head CT, EEG, Holter, cardiac enzymes, and carotid Doppler studies. Obviously, a complete work-up cannot be done in the ED.

5. Consider etiologies:

Seizure
TIA/Stroke
Hypovolemia
GI bleed
Heart block
Sick sinus syndrome
MI
PE
Hypoxia
Hypoglycemia
Psychiatric

Vasovagal syncope
Orthostatic hypotension
Carotid sinus hypersensitivity
Micturation syncope
Anemia
SVT
VT/VF
Pericardial Tamponade
IHSS
Aortic stenosis

6. Disposition: If an etiology cannot be attributed to findings, admission, or follow up with an internist for further studies will be necessary.

Throat Pain

Pharyngitis is most commonly caused by viruses, however, since strep infection can lead to rheumatic fever and glomerulonephritis, proper evaluation and treatment is essential. Absence of pharyngeal findings suggests possible epiglottitis or deep (fascial) space infection.

Streptococcal Pharyngitis: is impossible to diagnose on clinical grounds alone. Culture and/or rapid assay can be used to guide therapy, unless you decide to treat patients empirically.

Adults
- Penicillin G (benzathine) 1.2 Million Units IM.
- Penicillin VK 250mg PO QID for 10 days.
- E.E.S. 400mg PO TID for 10 days.

Less than 12 years
- Penicillin G (benzathine) 600,000 Units IM.
  (if less than 15kg then 300,000 Units IM).
- Penicillin 40mg/kg/day divided QID for 10 days.
- Erythromycin 40mg/kg/day divided TID for 10 days.

Non-streptococcal pharangitis: pathogens include:
- Gonococcal-Ceftriaxone 250mg IM.
- Meningococcus, Diphtheria, Mycoplasma/Legionella.
- Candida-immunocompromised patients.
- Mononucleosis-monospot may be helpful.
- Herpangina-painful ulcers (adeno/coxackievirus).

Deep Space Infections: are usually caused by strep, staph or H. flu, but may be polymicrobial/anaerobic in origin. Suspect in patient with throat pain but without pharyngeal or epiglottic findings.
- Peritonsillar Abscess: potential space under tonsillar capsule. Swelling and asymmetry of soft palate occur.
- Retro-pharyngeal Abscess: most common in children. Difficulty swallowing, neck pain. Lateral neck films show increased retro-pharyngeal space. Difficult to discern from epiglottitis.
- Prevertebral space infection.
- Para-pharyngeal Abscess: neck pain, fever, jaw pain, swelling of posterior pharynx.

Epiglottitis: usually presents with stridor, but should be considered in any patient with sufficient neck pain to cause drooling, neck extension(posturing) or a toxic or anxious look, or in patients with significant throat pain without pharyngeal findings. See Stridor page 64.

UTI

UTIs range from asymptomatic bacteruria to septic pyelonephritis. Treatment varies according to clinical and laboratory findings.

Symptoms and signs of lower UTI include lower abdominal pain, pelvic pain, dysuria, frequency, and fever. Children may present with anorexia, fever, or generalized fussiness. High fever, shaking chills, nausea, vomiting, back pain, flank pain or CVA tenderness suggest pyelonephritis.

Laboratory: Urinalysis (UA) with culture and sensitivity (C&S) is the mainstay of evaluation. Urine may be "clean catch" in patients able to perform the procedure however, elderly, obese, and infants may need to be catheterized.

Criteria for UTI:
>2-5 WBC/hpf in symptomatic women or asymptomatic men.
>5-10 WBC/hpf in women, regardless of symptoms.
Leukocyte Esterase-sensitive but not specific for pyuria.
Nitrate reaction-specific but not sensitive for bacteruria.

Treatment:

Asymptomatic bacteruria and uncomplicated lower UTI:
TMP/SMX Double strength (DS) PO BID for 3 days.
TMP/SMX (DS) PO BID for 7 days if pregnant.
(Avoid bactrim in the third trimester of pregnancy).
Phenazopyridine 200mg PO TID for 2 days bladder analgesic.

Children: Amoxicillin 40mg/kg/day divided TID PO for 10d.
Culture children but not adults.
Follow up with primary care in 1 week.

Persistent symptoms, repeat visit, uncomplicated pyelonephritis:
TMP/SMX (DS) PO BID for 14 days -or-
Ciprofloxacin 500mg PO BID for 14 days.
Urine culture, follow up 2wks.

Risk factors for STD, minimal pyuria/absent bacteria on UA:
Doxycycline 100mg PO BID for 10days or chlamydia culture.

Septic or Complicated Pyelonephritis:
Admit for IV antibiotics.

Vaginal Bleeding

1. Assess vitals and rule out life threatening hemorrhage. If older than ten and less than fifty, get a beta-hCG.
2. History: Age, PMH, meds, contraception, sexual activity, history of STD, IUD, ectopic pregnancy, or prior instrumentation.
   $G_{\#}P_{fpal}$: # pregnancies, full-term, pre-term, abortions, living.
   LNMP: first day of last menstrual period.
   Menstrual history: usual number of days between, days of bleeding, regular/irregular, heavy/light.
   Amount of bleeding: number of pads/tampons. One soaked pad or tampon usually indicates approximately 30cc of blood loss.
   If beta-positive:
   - EDC: estimated day of confinement. (-3mo + 7days from LNMP).
   - Weeks gestation: number of weeks and days.

3. Physical: orthostatics, general physical examination.
   Identify source of bleeding: per os, cervical, vaginal wall, rectal, urethral.
   Evaluate for cervical motion or adnexal tenderness. Using a gloved finger, determine in pregnant patients if the internal cervical os is open or closed. Do not insert any instruments beyond the external cervical os.

4. Laboratory: CBC, Type and screen for Rh status, PT/PTT.
   If urine beta positive get a quantitative beta-hCG.

5. Diagnosis

Beta Positive:

Ectopic Pregnancy: usually presents as abdominal pain with adnexal tenderness and uterine bleeding. See page 35.

Early Intrauterine Pregnancy

Abortion	Tissue	Bleeding	Cramping	Internal Os
Threatened	-	+	+/-	closed
Inevitable	-	+	+	open
Incomplete	+	+	+	open
Complete	+	+/-	+/-	closed
Missed	-	+/-	-	closed

Hydatidiform mole

Corpus luteum cyst,

Late Intrauterine Pregnancy: placenta previa, abruptio placentae and uterine rupture need to be ruled out. Transfer emergently to L&D.

Beta negative:

Cervical polyps or tumors	Trauma
Fibroid/Uterine cancer	Breakthrough bleeding
IUD	Infection

Dysfunctional uterine bleeding: essentially a diagnosis of exclusion.
If bleeding is severe, consult GYN. Follow up is essential.

Wounds and Lacerations

"I've always worked on the premise, hoping that what I did would be good today and good twenty or twenty five years from now."
Charles J. Johnson, on the design of White Tower restaurants.

1. History: mechanism and time of injury, last tetanus, allergies. Diabetes, keloid, collagen vascular disease, steroid use, chemo/RT.

2. Physical: description with drawing, type of injury: abrasion, puncture wound, avulsion, laceration-linear, flap, stellate (burst), tidy/untidy. Probe wound for FB, tendon, nerve, muscle, or vessel injury after anesthesia and prep, but do neuro exam prior to block.

3. Anesthesia: done before prep to minimize patient discomfort. Lidocaine 1% is a good local anesthetic. While epinephrine helps with hemostasis, it also impairs healing to some degree. **Never inject epinephrine into a digit, nose, ear or penis**. Local infiltration into the wound margins should be sufficient, however, digital and regional blocks may be helpful.

4. Exploration: examine carefully for any foreign body, ruptured tendons, severed nerves or blood vessels. Probe gently to detect if deep fascial spaces have been penetrated.

5. Preparation: done in three steps:
    Surgical scrub: prep skin around wound but not wound itself.
        Betadine, Chlorhexidine, others.
    Wound prep: cleanse wound itself.
        Saline, Shur-cleans, others.
    Irrigation: saline injection from 60cc syringe through an 18G IV.
        50-100cc/cm for most wounds is sufficient.

    If bleeding restarts after prep, apply direct pressure with gauze and elevate extremity. If bleeding continues, apply pressure longer. Sometimes a BP cuff or tourniquet applied proximally may help. Do not apply for long periods.

6. Repair: handle tissues gently, don't crush delicate edges.
    Apply new pair of sterile gloves.
    Drape to expose only the wound.
    Sharply remove any dead or devitalized tissue.
    Re-approximate any periosteum or fascia and close in a layered fashion using absorbable sutures. Muscles do not suture well and re-approximate well by themselves if the surrounding fascia is repaired, however, muscles of the face should be approximated and sutured to avoid deformity.
    Close skin with simple interrupted non-absorbable sutures. Divide the wound equally and place them equi-distant from the wound margin.

Wounds and Lacerations (Continued)

"Never put anything in a wound that you wouldn't put in your eye."
Richard Edlich, MD, PhD.

7. Suture Materials:

Absorbable	Non-absorbable
Chromic Gut	Polyester
Vicryl	Nylon
PDS	Prolene

8. Dressing: Apply a thin layer of antimicrobial ointment and cover with sterile gauze. Other options include Bismuth (Xeroform) gauze or simply leaving the wound uncovered. Splints should be used to temporarily immobilize repairs over joints.

9. Suture Removal:

Repair	Days
Scalp	6-7
Ears	3-5
Neck (post)	5-7
Extremities	7-10
(flexor surface)	7-10
(extensor surface)	10-14

Repair	Days
Face	3-5
Neck (ant)	3-5
Torso/Abdomen	6-8
Palms/Soles	7-14

10. Wound Care Instructions:
    1. Keep wound clean and dry. Wet dressings must be changed.
    2. Leave wound alone. In 24 hours (face) or 48 hours (others), remove dressing and inspect wound. Wash with mild soap or hydrogen peroxide, pat dry with clean towel or gauze, apply a thin layer of antimicrobial ointment and rebandage. This should be done three times a day for facial wounds and once daily for others.
    3. Don't soak wound or swim until sutures are removed.
    4. Return to _____ in ___days for wound check and in ___ days for suture removal.
    5. If any signs of infection develop: pain, pus, redness, swelling, red streaks, fever, return to the emergency department immediately.

11. Tetanus Prophylaxis:

Prior # of Shots	Clean wound	Other wounds
0-1	Toxoid	Toxoid + TIG
2	Toxoid	Toxoid only[1]
3	Nothing[2]	Nothing[3]
Unknown	Toxoid	Toxoid + TIG

Toxoid=0.5cc IM   TIG=Tetanus Immune Globulin 250-500 Units IM.

[1] If wound 24 hrs old give TIG as well.
[2] If last Tetanus >10 yrs old give Toxoid.
[3] If last tetanus >5 yrs old give Toxoid.

Wrist and Forearm

Injuries to the wrist and forearm most commonly result from a fall on an outstretched hand. They include distal radial and ulnar fractures, carpal fractures, and carpal dislocations.

1. History: mechanism of injury, direct blow vs. fall onto hand vs. hyperflexion vs. hyperextension of wrist. Time since injury, immobilization, prehospital treatment. Past injuries to wrist. Coexisting disease.

2. Physical: keep splinted. Document radial pulse, capillary refill, motor function, and sensory exam of fingers. Examine for an open fracture.

3. Radiology: (standard views)
   Forearm: AP and lateral. Wrist: AP and lateral.

Colles' fracture: distal radius fracture with dorsal displacement of the distal fragment. It is most common in the elderly. Look for median nerve injury. Fractures with significant displacement or angulation, with articular involvement or comminution should get ED ortho consultation. Minimally displaced or angulated fractures can be placed in a volar hand splint with RICE and ortho follow up in two or three days.

Smith's fracture: distal radius fracture with volar displacement of the distal fragment. It most commonly occurs from a fall with wrist flexed. Consultation in the ED or next day referral should be obtained.

Other fractures: include the Monteggia fracture, a proximal ulnar fracture associated with a dislocation of the radial head; the Galeazzi fracture, a fracture of the junction of the middle and distal third of the radius with an associated distal radioulnar joint dislocation; the Nightstick fracture, a fracture of distal ulna from direct blow i.e. arm held up to protect face; and Torus (buckle) or green-stick fractures which occur in children. Non-displaced or non-angulated fractures may be splinted for early follow up, but compartment syndrome can occur and ED consultation is advised.

Styloid fractures: are common and usually heal well.

Scaphoid fractures: are often difficult to see on x-rays and fracture should not be excluded on radiographic grounds alone. Any patient with snuff-box tenderness or pain on axial loading of the thumb should be immobilized for 2 weeks in a thumb spica and scheduled for repeat films. Other carpal fractures or dislocations should receive ED ortho consultation.

Wrist sprains: (x-ray negative) should be placed in a volar wrist splint with wrist in 30° of dorsiflexion with RICE and orthopedic follow-up in one week. Make sure the patient does not have snuff-box tenderness.

EKGs

1. Get old EKG for comparison.

2. Systematic Examination:

   Rhythm

   Rate

   Intervals

   PR < 0.21 seconds

   QRS < 0.12 seconds

   QT rate related

   Axis - 30° to + 120° or upright in I and aVF (0° to 90°).

   Then PQRST...

   P wave morphology

   Q waves

   R wave progression

   ST segments - elevation or depression

   T waves

Rate: each little box is 0.04 sec. 5 little boxes is 0.2 sec.

One beat per big box=300bpm, 2=150, 3=100, 4=75, 5=60, 6=50.

ST Segments:

Ischemia - depression

Infarction - elevation

Distribution of Infarction:

Anterior - precordial (V_2-V_6).

Inferior - II, III, aVF.

Lateral - I, aVL, V_5, V_6.

Posterior - reciprocal, large R or ST depression in V_1-V_2.

Index

Index